Management Issues in Schizophrenia

Management Issues in Schizophrenia

John M Kane

Chairman, Department of Psychiatry, Hillside Hospital

Professor of Psychiatry and Neuroscience
Albert Einstein College of Medicine
New York, USA

MARTIN DUNITZ

The cover painting is reproduced with the kind permission of Julia Burnett

First published in the United Kingdom in 2000 by
Martin Dunitz Ltd
The Livery House
7–9 Pratt Street
London NW1 0AE

Tel: +44 (0)207 482 2202
Fax: +44 (0)207 267 0159
E-mail: info@mdunitz.globalnet.co.uk
Website: http://www.dunitz.co.uk

A CIP record for this book is available from the British Library

ISBN 1-85317-940-X

Printed and bound in Italy by Printer Trento S.r.l.

Contents

Introduction

Schizophrenia remains one of the most challenging diseases in medicine. The disorder affects to varying degrees a range of functions including cognition, affect, behaviour, mood and motivation. As a result this disease can interfere with adaptation and achievement and robs people of many of the things that are taken for granted in day-to-day life.

Schizophrenia affects approximately 1% of the population and this lifetime prevalence appears to be similar throughout the world, though symptoms and course may vary from culture to culture. Since the illness usually begins in late adolescence or early adulthood critical aspects of emotional development, such as separation and individuation, may be interfered with. Since the disorder is often persistent or recurrent, long-term treatment is generally indicated. Full recovery occurs only in a small minority.

Although the aetiology and pathophysiology of schizophrenia have not been established, there are a number of important clues which should ultimately lead to further advances in treatment. Clearly, there is a strong genetic component; however, rates of discordance among monozygotic twins indicate that genetic vulnerability is only part of the picture. It may turn out that what we now label as schizophrenia is more than one disease, or a disease with a variety of aetiologic factors which play greater or lesser roles in any given individual.

The dopamine hypothesis has been of enormous value both in practical terms and in encouraging further research, as all currently available effective treatments for the psychosis intrinsic to schizophrenia have some degree of dopamine receptor blocking activity. It has also been shown that dopamine receptor agonists are capable of exacerbating signs and symptoms of schizophrenia, and some reports of increased dopamine receptor density in tissue of patients with schizophrenia obtained at autopsy also support the notion of some hyperactivity in dopaminergic systems. Some studies imaging living human brain using positron emission tomography (PET) or single photon emission computed tomography (SPECT) have also shown abnormalities in dopamine activity, though not all studies agree with these findings.

Despite the fact that the underlying cause of this disease has not been identified, important advances have been made in treatment, both pharmacologic and psychosocial. Major challenges remain in knowledge transfer to clinicians and patients as well as to families. The success of these efforts affect treatment application and treatment acceptance. All too often advances in treatment research and development are not adequately translated into day-to-day clinical management.

The treatment of schizophrenia is further complicated by the persisting stigma and lack of information associated with mental illness, particularly psychotic disorders such as schizophrenia. This directly and indirectly influences many aspects of the management of this disease, from early diagnosis and treatment to inadequate or inconsistent community services, as well as the ability of patients to reintegrate into the community.

The fact that schizophrenia has different phases over its course also adds to the challenge of clinical management because each phase can require a specific management strategy and each treatment decision must also be influenced by the patient's wishes, personality, way of thinking, family environment, psychosocial supports and (in many cases) economic resources and regional care resources.

An additional challenge in the management of this illness is the need to integrate different treatment modalities in the care of a given individual, recognizing that different components will be provided by different people or even different programmes. The need to share information and planning is often addressed more in theory than in practice. Over the coming years advances in information technology will no doubt facilitate this process.

The costs associated with schizophrenia — both direct, in terms of treatment costs, and indirect, in terms of lost productivity — are staggering. A disease affecting only 1% of the population accounts for a much higher proportion of overall disability costs when compared with many other diseases.

Diagnosis, course and outcome

Diagnosis of schizophrenia

One of the most important aspects of schizophrenia is the fact that it affects so many different domains of functioning, varying from individual to individual and to some extent within individuals over time. Although there are core features of schizophrenia that affect perception (hallucinations), cognition (attention, working memory, etc.), motivation (avolition), inferential reasoning (delusions) and affect (blunted or inappropriate), there is no pathognomonic sign or symptom of the disease.

Though disagreement still exists as to the boundaries of this disorder, both the World Health Organization and the American Psychiatric Association (APA) have developed criterion-based nosologies which satisfy modern-day requirements for validity and reliability.[1,2] Structured interviews are available which facilitate research,[3–5] but can also be helpful to clinicians in providing a standardized systematic format for eliciting the signs and symptoms necessary to make a diagnosis (in addition to excluding other diagnoses or recognizing co-morbid conditions that might affect course, response to treatment and outcome).

While there are some differences between the WHO criteria (Table 1) and the APA criteria (Table 2) they are overall quite similar and considerable cross-communication took place in their development. The main differences between the two systems relate to the duration requirement. The DSM definition requires a 6-month duration, whereas ICD-10 requires a

Table 1 *ICD diagnostic criteria.*[1]

At least one of the symptoms (a)–(d) or at least two of the symptoms (e)–(i) should have been present during a period of *a month or more*:
(a) thought echo, thought insertion or withdrawal, and thought broadcasting
(b) delusions of control, influence or passivity, clearly referred to body or limb movements or specific thoughts, actions or sensations; delusional perception
(c) hallucinatory voices giving a running commentary on the patient's behaviour, or discussing the patient among themselves, or other types of hallucinatory voices coming from some part of the body
(d) persistent delusions of other kinds that are culturally inappropriate and completely impossible, such as religious or political identity, or superhuman powers and abilities
(e) persistent hallucinations in any modality, accompanied either by fleeting or half-formed delusions without clear affective component, or by persistent overvalued ideas, or occurring every day for weeks or months on end
(f) breaks or interpolations in the train of thought, resulting in incoherence or irrelevant speech, or neologisms
(g) catatonic behavior, such as excitement, posturing, or waxy flexibility, negativism, mutism and stupor
(h) 'negative' symptoms such as marked apathy, paucity of speech and blunting or incongruity of emotional responses, usually resulting in social withdrawal and lowering of social performance; it must be clear that they are not due to depression or to neuroleptic medication
(i) a significant and consistent change in the overall quality of some aspects of personal behaviour, manifest as loss of interest, aimlessness, idleness, a self-absorbed attitude and social withdrawal.

1-month duration. In addition DSM requires a deterioration in functioning which is not required by ICD-10. As a result the DSM-IV definition is somewhat narrower.

Table 2 *DSM-IV diagnostic criteria.*[2]

A *Characteristic symptoms.* At least two of the following symptoms, each present for significant portion of the time during a 1-month period:
(a) delusions
(b) hallucinations
(c) disorganized speech (e.g. frequent derailment or incoherence)
(d) grossly disorganized or catatonic behaviour
(e) negative symptoms, i.e. affective flattening, alogia or avolition

F *Social/occupational dysfunction.* For a significant portion of the time since the onset of the disturbance, one or more major areas of functioning such as work, interpersonal relationships or self-care are markedly below the level achieved prior to the onset

G *Duration.* Continuous signs of the disturbance persist for at least 6 months. This 6-month period must include at least 1 month of symptoms that meet criterion A and may include periods of prodromal and residual symptoms. During these prodromal or residual periods the signs of the disturbance may be manifested by only negative symptoms or two or more symptoms listed in criterion A present in attenuated form

H *Schizoaffective and mood disorder exclusion.* Schizoaffective and mood disorders have been ruled out because either (1) no major depressive, manic or mixed episodes have occurred concurrently with the active-phase symptoms; or (2) if mood episodes have occurred during active-phase symptoms, their total duration has been brief relative to the duration of the active and residual periods

I *Substance/general medical condition exclusion.* The disturbance is not due to the direct physiological effects of a substance (e.g. drug of abuse, a medication) or a general medical condition

J *Relationship to a pervasive developmental disorder.* If there is a history of autistic disorder or another pervasive developmental disorder, the additional diagnosis of schizophrenia is made only if prominent delusions or hallucinations are also present for at least 1 month.

There has been a long history of dividing schizophrenia into different subtypes (e.g. paranoid) as well as categorizing its manifestations (e.g. positive, negative, disorganized). The clinical usefulness of these distinctions should be viewed from a number of perspectives. For example, to what extent do these categories influence patient case finding, treatment response and course of illness — in other words, what impact do they have on day-to-day clinical management decisions?

Positive symptoms are more likely to lead to acute treatment and overall tend to respond better to available pharmacotherapies. On the other hand, negative symptoms and cognitive dysfunction are more relevant in predicting psychosocial and vocational adjustment. One of the greatest challenges in working with patients and families is setting realistic goals and expectations for treatment response and overall functional ability. Understanding the implications of different symptom patterns and subtypes in this context is particularly helpful. However, our ability to treat such phenomena as negative symptoms and cognitive dysfunction successfully, though improving, still has a long way to go.

It is important to recognize that in some situations negative symptoms can be secondary rather than primary. Parkinsonian side-effects such as akinesia can lead to diminished affect, spontaneity and motivation. Depression or demoralization can mimic some aspects of negative symptoms and some patients may be uncommunicative and withdrawn with psychomotor retardation secondary to positive symptoms. Environmental deprivation such as chronic institutionalization or isolated living circumstances in the community could also contribute to apathy and withdrawal. Some aspects of cognitive impairment, particularly in memory, could be attributable to anticholinergic medications.

The concept of 'deficit symptoms' was an attempt to establish a category of negative symptoms that not only persisted, but were not attributable to other causes.[6]

Course and outcome

The course of schizophrenia can be loosely divided into three phases: prodromal, early–acute and late phase–chronic. The timing and definition of the prodromal phase is the most poorly defined. Some aspects of schizophrenia are apparent many years before the psychotic signs and symptoms become manifest. Mild abnormalities in psychomotor activity, motor coordination, social skills and cognitive function have been identified in individuals who went on to receive a diagnosis of schizophrenia.[7–9] Although sometimes these abnormalities are described as premorbid, if they are actually early manifestations of the disease they may more appropriately be labelled as prodromal, even though this phase may last for over a decade. Not all of these abnormalities are seen in every individual who goes on to develop schizophrenia, and some may exhibit none of them. Drawing conclusions in this context is particularly difficult, since in an area such as cognitive functioning it is impossible to know what level an individual would have achieved without the changes brought about by a putative neurodevelopmental disorder. Data that support the notion of early cognitive effects are based on group comparisons of subjects who went on to develop schizophrenia compared with appropriately matched normal controls. In addition, these early abnormalities may not be specific to schizophrenia.

In future the management of schizophrenia might include primary prevention for subjects at high risk and secondary prevention for individuals who are beginning to show what we might call prodromal phase symptomatology.

The prodromal phase includes the period when non-specific signs and symptoms emerge that differ from the person's previous characteristics and ultimately affect functioning. The onset of these symptoms is often gradual, but the time course can vary enormously: some estimates suggest an average duration of 2–4 years, but with an extremely broad range. Late prodromal signs and symptoms include irritability, depressed mood, sleep disturbance, suspiciousness, ideas of reference, odd behaviour and blunted affect. None of these symptoms is specific; they can occur in other disorders, or be transient and not clinically significant. However, some portion of these symptoms precede the onset of full-blown psychosis in most individuals who ultimately receive a diagnosis of schizophrenia.

Early intervention

The duration of these prodromal symptoms — particularly the duration of untreated psychotic symptoms — may be associated with poorer response to treatment once it is initiated. On the other hand, it is possible that individuals with a more insidious onset and those who are reluctant to seek treatment have a poorer prognosis in general.

Some studies have reported significant correlations between these variables;[10] however, others have not,[11,12] and controlled comparisons would be necessary to eliminate confounds. The only study that provided appropriate controls for comparison was by May and colleagues in which some patients were randomly assigned to conditions other than medication treatment.[13] These individuals had a poorer course over the next 3–4 years, despite ultimately receiving pharmacotherapy. This suggests that a lengthy (in this case 6 months) delay in initiating medication can have an impact on outcome. Other studies have examined shorter delays (e.g. 4–6 weeks) in treatment initiative and have found no measurable sequelae.

A number of efforts are under way to improve early detection and to facilitate earlier treatment intervention. Clearly from a psychosocial, psychodynamic and possibly biologic perspective, the duration of untreated psychosis should be reduced as much as possible.

Investigators in several countries have implemented large-scale programs designed to facilitate early detection of psychosis and early intervention. These efforts have highlighted the potential value of community and professional education, improving patient access and designing specialty programmes to meet the particular needs of patients and families during this phase of illness.

Falloon et al. conducted a pilot study suggesting that with appropriate early identification of prodromal signs and intervention the incidence of florid episodes of psychosis could be reduced.[14] The programme involved close liaison between family practitioners and mental health professionals who were specifically trained in management of patients during this phase of illness (including pharmacotherapy, psychoeducation of patients and families, stress management and case management). This program employed a ten-question screening instrument (10-QS) (Table 3)

Table 3 *A ten-question screening (10-QS). From Falloon et al.*[14]

1. How have you been sleeping in the past week? Any difficulties getting to sleep? Waking early?
2. Have you lost your appetite recently? Weight loss of 2 kg or more?
3. Have you experienced loss of energy or interests recently?
4. Have you been worrying a lot about everyday problems?
5. Have you had difficulty concentrating on reading or watching television?
6. Have you been more forgetful than usual? How do you see the future? Do you ever feel that life is not worth living? Have you ever felt you would like to end it all?
7. Have you any odd habits, like checking or cleaning more than other people?
8. Do you ever have attacks of palpitations, sweating, shaking or dizziness accompanied by feelings of intense fear?
9. Has anybody commented that your speech has become odd or difficult to understand?
10. Have you ever had the experience of hearing people's voices speaking when nobody seems to be around?

and eight early-warning signs of schizophrenia derived from the prodromal signs outlined in DSM-III (Table 4). These tools were used by family practitioners to screen for individuals who should receive further assessment by mental health professionals. The initial consultation with a specialist was carried out jointly with the family practitioner or community nurse whenever possible. Using an analysis of new cases of florid psychosis over a specified interval in a semirural area with a population of 35 000 people, the authors found a reduction in incidence estimates after this programme had been implemented. As the authors suggested the results must be interpreted with caution, but were certainly encouraging and helped to establish a model for further efforts.

McGorry and colleagues developed an early psychosis prevention and intervention centre (EPPIC) in Melbourne, Australia.[15] In addition to providing specialized care to adolescents and young adults experiencing the first onset of a psychotic illness, the centre has developed community education activities to increase awareness of the nature of psychosis in young people and to promote early recognition and referral. Preliminary reports suggest significant improvements in symptomatic and functional outcome. Larsen et al. have reported on an early intervention

Table 4 *Prodromal signs checklist. From Falloon et al.*[14]

Onset of one of the following without explanation:
• Marked peculiar behaviour
• Inappropriate, or loss of, expression of feelings
• Speech that is difficult to follow
• Marked lack of speech and thoughts
• Marked preoccupation with odd ideas
• Ideas of reference — things have special meanings
• Persistent feelings of unreality
• Changes in the way things appear, sound or smell

programme in Norway which also involves educational efforts targeted at primary-care health professionals and extensive community education.[16] Cornblatt et al. have developed a specialized clinic for recognition and prevention of psychological problems (RAPP) at Hillside Hospital in New York, which focuses on individuals experiencing potentially prodromal states and is attempting to develop predictors of who goes on to develop more significant psychopathology in order to help establish when pharmacologic intervention is appropriate.[17] Ultimately, these programmes will help to inform clinicians as to the best therapeutic options.

There are no clear-cut guidelines as to what forms of treatment are most effective. Antipsychotic drug therapy during the prodromal phase has become more feasible with the introduction of a new generation of medications which are much less likely to cause neurologic side-effects such as dystonia, drug-induced parkinsonism, akathisia and tardive dyskinesia. Previously concerns about these adverse effects, particularly tardive dyskinesia, would have been a major impediment to an intervention strategy that preceded a diagnosis of schizophrenia. On the other hand, weight gain has emerged as a real concern with most of the newer drugs, particularly in adolescents and young adults.[18]

The most important recommendation at present is to foster and facilitate the referral to experienced mental health professionals of individuals who may be experiencing a prodrome of psychosis. Psychotherapy, stress management and development of a therapeutic alliance and careful follow-up will at least permit the earliest possible intervention once it is clearly indicated. This alone would be an important step towards reducing the delay in treating first psychotic episodes.

Acute phase

The early acute phase describes the emergence of psychotic signs and symptoms sufficient to warrant a diagnosis of schizophrenia. The severity and pattern of symptoms can vary enormously, but it usually includes positive symptoms such as delusions or hallucinations and/or disorganized behaviour which precipitates treatment referral and often hospitalization. The average age at which this phase begins is the early 20s, with a significantly younger age of onset for males.[19] The reasons for this have not been established, but this sex difference is seen in many other neuropsychiatric conditions.

There is no clear delineation as to when the early acute phase ends and the chronic phase begins. Response to treatment in the first psychotic episode is usually good, with over 70% of patients achieving a full remission of psychotic signs and symptoms within a period of 3–4 months and often more rapidly.[20] However, follow-up studies suggest that within five years 75–80% of patients will have relapsed. Medication is the single most important factor in reducing the risk of relapse, but many patients do not wish to continue taking medication on a long-term basis. It is hoped that the new-generation medications will help to improve this situation.

Late phase

A late phase chronic period is seen in patients who show significant deterioration in functional ability, compared with their level of psychosocial, academic or vocational adjustment prior to the onset of late prodromal phase or acute phase illness. The time at which this occurs varies, but it is often within the first 5–10 years of illness. The course of illness in terms of symptom patterns also varies considerably; negative symptoms may become more prominent over time and relapses can occur with varying frequency and intensity (influenced to an important degree by treatment management). Long-term follow-up studies (over 20 years) suggest that many patients achieve a stable plateau where no further deterioration occurs and the signs and symptoms of the illness are less florid.[21] However, a substantial subgroup of patients respond poorly to available treatments and experience persistent psychotic signs and symptoms.[22] Few patients are unresponsive or poorly responsive to treatment during their initial episode of psychosis, so some process occurs that reduces medication responsiveness over time in a subgroup of patients; the factors contributing to this course have not been identified.

Unfortunately, the prediction of outcome in schizophrenia is difficult, complicating our ability to inform patients and families as to what to expect and complicating our attempts to establish realistic long-term goals. It is important, however, not to give up hope of further improvement even in the most severely ill patients, as demonstrated by the surprising impact of clozapine in many such individuals.[23] It is also hoped that advances in our ability to foster treatment compliance and reduce relapse rates could significantly improve long-term outcome.

Other factors that can influence course and outcome include availability of psychosocial support and treatment, social skills training, work opportunities, family environment, co-morbid conditions such as substance abuse or depression, and personality factors.

New-generation antipsychotic medications

Antipsychotic medications are by far the most effective treatment for schizophrenia. These drugs have revolutionalized patient care since their introduction in the 1950s. However, medication cannot be given in isolation and an array of other psychosocial, family and vocational therapies should also be applied when appropriate. The timing, sequencing and duration of specific interventions will vary from patient to patient and from one phase of illness to another, but the thoughtful integration of these approaches is essential to optimizing long-term outcome.

Chlorpromazine was the first antipsychotic to be introduced into clinical practice after serendipitous observations regarding its 'tranquillizing' effects, which ultimately proved to be almost uniquely antipsychotic. Its introduction in the 1950s was followed by the introduction of an array of different classes of antipsychotic drugs (at that time also referred to as 'neuroleptic' drugs, since they were associated with a degree of extrapyramidal side-effects — or drug-induced parkinsonism). Although these drugs differed in their chemical structure, neuroreceptor binding profile and adverse effects, they were all associated with blockade of dopamine D_2 receptors, contributing to the establishment of the dopamine hypothesis. These medications were generally thought to be interchangeable in terms of efficacy. In 100 studies comparing the effectiveness of chlorpromazine, thioridazane, and trifluoperazine with that of other drugs listed in Table 5 (excluding clozapine and other 'atypical' or new-generation medications such as risperidone, olanzapine and quetiapine),

Table 5 *Typical doses and estimated relative potency of conventional antipsychotic drugs. The equivalent dose is the number of milligrams of the drug required for the dose to be equivalent to the doses of the other drugs in the table (e.g. 100 mg of chlorpromazine is equivalent to 2 mg of haloperidol). Relative potency may not be the same at higher dosages as at lower ones.*

Drug	Equivalent dose* (mg)	Usual total daily dose: Short-term therapy (mg/day)	Usual total daily dose: Maintenance therapy (mg/day)
Phenothiazines			
Chlorpromazine	100	200–1000	50–400
Thioridazine	100	200–800	50–400
Mesoridazine	50	100–400	25–200
Acetophenazine	20	60–150	40–80
Prochlorperazine	15	60–200	20–60
Perphenazine	10	12–64	8–24
Trifluoperazine	5	10–60	4–30
Triflupromazine	25	30–150	20–100
Fluphenazine	2	5–50	1–15
Thioxanthenes			
Thiothixene	5	10–60	6–30
Chlorprothixene	100	50–600	50–400
Butyrophenones			
Haloperidol	2	5–50	1–15
Dibenzoxazepines			
Loxapine	10	20–160	10–60
Dihydroindolones			
Molindone	10	40–225	15–100

Table 5 *Contd.*

Drug	Equivalent dose* (mg)	Usual total daily dose: Short-term therapy (mg/day)	Usual total daily dose: Maintenance therapy (mg/day)
Long-acting injectable preparations			
Fluphenazine decanoate			6–100 mg every 2–4 wk
Haloperidol decanoate			50–200 mg every 4 wk
Flupenthixol decanoate			20–300 mg every 2–4 wk
Zuclopenthixol decanoate			200–400 mg every 2–4 wk
Pipothiazine palmitate			50–100 mg every 4 wk

only one study reported a significant difference and this would be expected by chance.[24,25] It is important to recognize, however, that these findings are based on group comparisons and do not necessarily mean that an individual patient might not respond better to one drug than another.

The conventional antipsychotic agents have been associated with a number of problems. Perhaps most importantly, they produce a relatively high incidence of neurologic adverse effects ranging from acute dystonia to akathisia and akinesia, and more infrequent (but much more serious) effects such as tardive dyskinesia and neuroleptic malignant syndrome (Table 6). Conventional antipsychotics therefore often required the administration of concomitant (usually anticholinergic antiparkinsonian) medication to prevent or alleviate the parkinsonian or dystonic reactions. The risk of tardive dyskinesia often led to hesitation in recommending long-term treatment, particularly for patients in relative remission, or those who had experienced only one psy-

Table 6 *Extrapyramidal side-effects. The incidence rates are for conventional antipsychotic drugs.*

	Incidence	Description	Differential diagnosis
Akathisia	20–25%	Subjective sense of restlessness or jitteriness Objective restlessness: pacing, agitation Can lead to aggressive or self-injurious behaviour	Anxiety: psychotic agitation Substance abuse Alcohol withdrawal Benzodiazepine withdrawal
Akinesia	15–35%	Diminished spontaneous movements or gestures Constricted affect Slowed movements Feeling slowed down or lacking in motivation	Depression Negative symptoms Demoralization
Dystonia	2–10%	Muscle cramps or spasms Sustained muscle contractions; often affects muscles of head and neck, can affect speech or swallowing	Dissociative phenomena Malingering

chotic episode. The use of anticholinergic drugs carries its own side-effect burden, including possible impairment in memory functions. Not only are these side-effects subjectively distressing, but they can also be associated with behavioural and functional disturbances such as the restlessness or agitation associated with akathisia — which when misdiagnosed can lead to inappropriate additional pharmacotherapy — or the lack of spontaneity, blunted affect or motor retardation associated with akinesia which can mimic some aspects of negative symptoms. Side-effects such as tardive dyskinesia (and more rarely tardive dystonia) in their severe forms can be disfiguring and disabling, but even in their milder forms can add to the stigma and social embarrassment associated with the illness. Neuroleptic malignant syndrome is potentially life-threatening if not appropriately diagnosed and adequately treated. Conventional antipsychotic drugs are also associated with a variety of other potential side-effects to varying degrees involving almost all organ systems. Conventional drugs are not always effective and tend to be more effective against positive rather than negative symptoms or cognitive dysfunction. In addition, non-compliance rates have been high and a substantial subgroup of patients relapse despite taking medication.

It is against this background that a new generation of so-called 'atypical' medications was introduced. Clozapine, the prototype, was not a new drug in terms of development, but its use had been limited because of an increased risk of agranulocytosis. Although some of its novel properties, such as a low incidence of extrapyramidal side-effects, minimal prolactin elevation and superior clinical effectiveness, had been described, it was not until clear superiority in carefully selected treatment-refractory patients was demonstrated that clozapine was brought into widespread clinical use along with careful monitoring of white blood cell counts (following the recognition that clozapine-induced agranulocytosis was readily reversible if early detection took place).[23]

Clozapine has a broad array of receptor-binding affinities, including serotonin 5-HT_{2a}, 5-HT_{2c}, 5-HT_6, α_1 and α_2 adrenergic, M_1 muscarinic, H_1 histaminergic and D_4 (and to a lesser extent D_1 D_2 and D_3) dopamine receptors. The role of specific receptor effects, combinations or ratios of receptor effects which account for clozapine's novel properties has yet to be firmly established, although emphasis has been given to serotonergic and adrenergic mechanisms in various hypotheses. In addition, findings with regard to receptor effects differ between in vitro and in vivo studies and from one brain region to another. Therefore, much remains to be learned about the mechanisms of specific drug effects.

Considerable effort has gone into replicating clozapine's novel properties by producing compounds with structural similarity (e.g. olanzapine) and/or compounds that combine specific receptor effects (e.g. risperidone, sertindole, quetiapine, ziprasidone). Amisulpride is also considered to have some atypical properties yet its binding profile differs in many respects from other drugs in this category.

Figure 1 provides an overview of the new-generation drugs and their receptor-binding profiles. Although these drugs differ from each other, in general they have relatively high affinities for dopamine D_2 and serotonin 5-HT_2 receptors. As a class they produce fewer parkinsonian side-effects and preliminary results suggest less tardive dyskinesia as well.

Amisulpride

Amisulpride's binding profile is highly selective for D_2 and D_3 dopamine receptors. It demonstrates no affinity for serotonergic, histaminergic or α adrenergic receptors. The low incidence of extrapyramidal side-effects (EPS) associated with amisulpride is probably attributable to a degree of limbic specificity despite its selective dopamine antagonism.[26]

Amisulpride has been shown to be as effective as haloperidol in the treatment of positive symptoms,[27,28] and potentially more effective in the treatment of negative symptoms, where low doses may be sufficient.[29] Elevated serum prolactin is associated with amisulpride, and can cause sexual dysfunction.[30]

With increasing dose the incidence of EPS does increase, but at low doses the compound also acts as an antagonist at presynaptic autoreceptors,[26] thereby enhancing the release of dopamine, which may account for its helpful effects on negative symptoms. Amisulpride can cause insomnia, anxiety, agitation, constipation, nausea and dry mouth. Systematic data on the incidence of tardive dyskinesia are not available. Weight gain occurs to a slight degree.

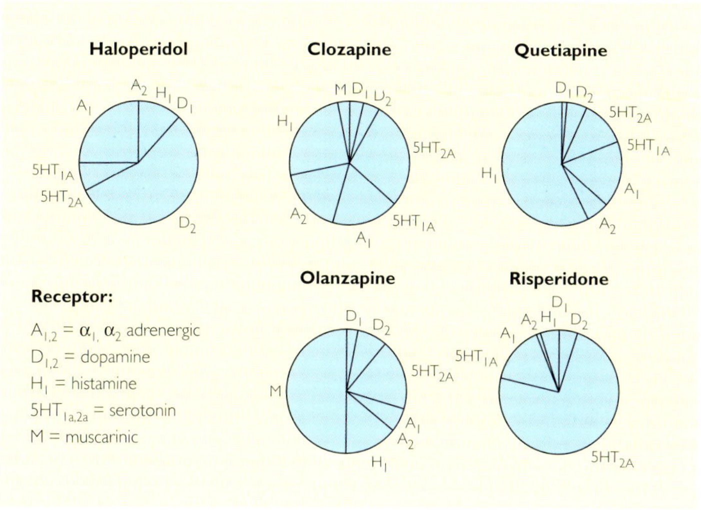

Figure 1 *Receptor binding characteristics of haloperidol and some atypical antipsychotics.*

Risperidone

Risperidone's efficacy was established in a number of double-blind, controlled trials of acutely psychotic patients, in which it was found to be superior to haloperidol on some measures.[31,32] Doses of 4–6 mg per day are recommended for most patients; there is no evidence that doses above 6 mg are associated with better response, but they do produce a higher incidence of EPS. Risperidone has been shown to be helpful in some patients who failed to respond to other drugs,[33–35] but it does not appear to be as effective in treatment-refractory patients as clozapine when all available data are considered. Risperidone is associated with sedation and orthostatic hypotension, so gradual dose titration is recommended during the initial phase of treatment. Risperidone is associated with significant prolactin elevation, although the occurrence of clinically significant immediate sequelae appears to be low. Weight gain is seen in a proportion of patients, but is less pronounced than with clozapine or olanzapine. The incidence of tardive dyskinesia appears to be significantly lower than with conventional antipsychotics.

Olanzapine

Olanzapine has some similarities with clozapine in its chemical structure and its pharmacologic profile.[36] Doses of 10–20 mg are generally recommended. In comparative trials olanzapine was shown to be at least as effective as haloperidol and in some studies superior, particularly on measures of negative and depressive symptoms.[37–39]

In long-term comparisons olanzapine has been shown to be at least as effective as haloperidol and possibly superior in the prevention of relapse.[40] In one 6-month study olanzapine was superior to risperidone in preventing exacerbations during the continuation phase of treatment.[40]

Olanzapine has been shown to be helpful in some refractory patients,[41–43] but in a controlled comparison with chlorpromazine in refractory patients olanzapine was not superior.[44]

At low and moderate doses olanzapine produced no more EPS than was observed in the placebo-treated comparison group, but at higher doses it was associated with significantly more akathisia than placebo (but less than observed with haloperidol). Olanzapine is associated with a slight to modest dose-related prolactin elevation, and weight gain can be a significant problem. In a long-term comparison with haloperidol, olanzapine was associated with a significantly lower incidence of tardive dyskinesia.[38]

Quetiapine

In controlled comparisons quetiapine was shown to be superior to placebo and as effective as haloperidol and chlorpromazine.[45–47]

The incidence of EPS with quetiapine appears to be the lowest of the new-generation drugs, although direct comparisons are not available between all of the new drugs. The incidence of tardive dyskinesia in patients undergoing continuation treatment was much lower than would be expected with conventional antipsychotic drugs.[48] Quetiapine is not associated with prolactin elevation and the risk of weight gain appears to be lower than for olanzapine and similar to that for risperidone. In a study of partial responders quetiapine 600 mg/day was associated with a significantly higher proportion of patients achieving a 20% reduction in total Positive And Negative Syndrome Scale (PANSS) scores than observed with haloperidol 20 mg/day.[49] Dizziness and orthostatic hypotension can occur during treatment implementation and a slow dosage increase is therefore recommended.

Sertindole

Sertindole has been shown to be as effective as haloperidol and superior to placebo in short-term trials.[50–51] A long-term study comparing it with haloperidol showed significantly lower rehospitalization rates with sertindole.[52] Sertindole is associated with a very low incidence of EPS and is the only drug to date that has been compared with multiple fixed doses of a conventional drug;[50] it was associated with significantly fewer EPS than even 4 mg/day of haloperidol, supporting the conclusion that the superiority of the new-generation drugs in producing few EPS is not explainable by high doses of the comparator drug.

Sertindole has been associated with one unusual side-effect, reduction in ejaculatory volume. The major problem with sertindole has been a prolongation in the QT_c interval of the electrocardiogram (ECG).[50] Although the clinical relevance of this is still debated, sertindole is not currently actively marketed.

Ziprasidone

Ziprasidone combines D_2, D_4 and 5-HT_2 antagonism, but also acts as a 5-HT_{1c} agonist and inhibits norepinephrine and serotonin reuptake. It has been shown to be superior to placebo and as effective as haloperidol in acute treatment and continuation treatment.[53–55] In a 1-year placebo-controlled maintenance trial in chronic but stable in-patients ziprasidone showed effectiveness in preventing psychotic relapse and improving negative symptoms.[56] This study is important in demonstrating that improvement in negative symptoms is not merely attributable to withdrawal from a conventional antipsychotic drug.

The risk of EPS was only slightly greater than that seen with placebo in both acute and long-term trials. Ziprasidone is associated with the least amount of weight gain of the new drugs.[18] There is no significant prolactin elevation, but there is some degree of QT_c prolongation. Data on the risk of tardive dyskinesia are not yet available, but the low propensity to produce EPS suggests a reduced risk of tardive dyskinesia.

Zotepine

Zotepine combines dopamine (D_1, D_2, D_3 and D_4) and serotonin (5-HT_{2a} and 5-HT_{2c}) antagonism with α_1 adrenergic and H_1 histaminergic receptor antagonism. The drug has been shown to be effective in short-term trials against haloperidol and placebo.[57–59] In a 6-month trial zotepine was superior to placebo in prevention of relapse.[60] In a study of patients with predominant negative symptoms zotepine produced greater improvement than haloperidol.[61]

Zotepine produces significantly fewer EPS than haloperidol. It is associated in a dose-related fashion with sedation, transient elevation in liver enzymes, and seizures. It can also produce postural hypotension.

Conclusion

The new-generation antipsychotic agents are a major advance in treating schizophrenia. They are associated with significantly fewer neurologic side-effects, the major disadvantage of conventional medications. In a number of studies advantages are seen over conventional medications in negative symptoms, and in fewer studies in positive symptoms. The drugs are effective in relapse prevention and may be associated with lower relapse rates, though available data are limited. Measurements of cognitive function suggest improvement with many of the newer agents, though much remains to be done in establishing their long-term functional impact. In addition, there are data supporting the value of new medications in improving outcome in a subgroup of patients who have been poor or partial responders to conventional antipsychotic therapy.

New-generation antipsychotic drugs have also been shown to be more helpful in alleviating symptoms of anxiety and depression which are frequently observed in patients with schizophrenia. In addition, several studies suggest advantages in reducing hostility and aggression and possibly suicidal behaviour as well.

The disadvantages of the newer drugs include the lack of availability of long-acting preparations, and the scarcity of short-acting intramuscular agents. In addition, the new drugs are associated to varying degrees with significant weight gain which can be troubling and poses serious health risks if it persists.

Treatment of acute psychotic episodes

Managing the first episode

Treating the first episode of schizophrenia is particularly critical because to some extent it sets the stage for subsequent treatment and establishes early patient and family knowledge of and attitudes toward the illness. In addition, it is possible that successful early intervention is associated with better prognosis. Most studies have found that patients receiving their first treatment for schizophrenia have already been ill with psychotic signs and symptoms for many weeks or months (Table 7). The reasons for the delay in seeking or accepting treatment are many and varied. Since the onset of this illness is often in late adolescence or early adulthood, frequently a time of emotional turmoil, families may be uncertain as to what constitutes a 'pathological' situation. Families may also consciously or unconsciously hesitate to recognize or acknowledge the seriousness of the problem because of the fear of what it might represent and the stigma associated with mental illness.

In some cases early contacts with primary-care physicians or even mental health professionals do not lead to the appropriate diagnosis. Since the early diagnosis can be difficult it is important that health-care providers in general (and ideally teachers, the clergy and ultimately the public at large) should have some training and familiarity with the early signs of this illness. Access to adequate psychiatric resources is also essential and many psychiatric hospitals or clinics are not equipped to deal specifically with the needs and challenges involved in managing the first episode.

Table 7 *Treatment delay in schizophrenia.*

Author	Location	Sample size	Diagnostic criteria	Treatment delay (weeks)
Johnstone et al. (1986)[62]	London	253	ICD-9	26% > 52
Birchwood et al. (1993)[63]	Birmingham	128	ICD-9	30
Loebel et al. (1992)[10]	New York	70	RDC*	52
Haas and Sweeney (1992)[64]	New York	71	DSM-IIIR	99
Haffner et al. (1993)[19]	Germany	267	ICD-9	110
Beiser et al. (1993)[65]	Vancouver	72	DSM-III	56
McGorry and Singh (1995)[66]	Melbourne	60	DSM-III R	74
Larsen et al. (1998)[16]	Norway	43	DSM-III R	114
Craig et al. (2000)[11]	New York	155	DSM-IV	14

*Research Diagnostic Criteria

Treatment delivered in a setting with many chronically ill patients can be frightening and unnecessarily demoralizing to patients at this stage of the illness, and may contribute to high rates of discontinuing treatment. Psychosocial treatment and psychoeducation should be provided as soon as possible to patients, families or significant others. The approach should be tailored to the special needs of people experiencing their first episode, and whenever possible should be provided by people who have experience working with this population.

Accurate diagnosis of the first episode is essential since a misdiagnosis could lead to long-term treatment with inappropriate medication and a variety of potential adverse effects. In some cases the differential diagnosis (e.g. affective illnesses with psychotic features) can be difficult and requires a longitudinal perspective. In such cases clinicians must guard against premature conclusions and ensure the necessary observation and documentation of subsequent course and treatment response to confirm the diagnosis.

The first episode may be acute or insidious and delineating the prodrome from actual onset can be difficult. The insidious onset may indicate a poorer prognosis. In the differential diagnosis substance abuse is also an important consideration and urine screening tests should be conducted in patients presenting with a first-episode psychosis.

A variety of medical illnesses can present with or lead to psychotic signs and symptoms and although these cases are rare it is critical to exclude them (Table 8).

Table 8 *Medical conditions to be excluded when evaluating a first-episode psychosis.*

Toxic drug reaction
Endocrine disorders
Metabolic disorders
Epilepsy (particularly temporal lobe)
CNS neoplasm
Huntington's disease
System lupus erythematosus
Neurosyphilis
Wilson's disease

Treatment implementation

Once the diagnosis has been made treatment should be initiated as rapidly as possible along with education for patient and family as to the nature of the illness, available treatments, their benefits and risks and some discussion of the longer-term treatment plan. Clinicians need to use their judgment as to the timing of these discussions, based on clinical state, family attitudes, and so on.

The decision as to what medication and what dose to use should take into account the special vulnerabilities of first-episode patients both psychologically and pharmacologically. In general patients receiving antipsychotic drugs for the first time require considerably lower doses than more chronic patients and are sensitive to the neurologic side-effects such as dystonia, akathisia and drug-induced parkinsonism (Table 9). Although some clini-

Table 9 *Dosage recommendations for new antipsychotic drugs. Dosage requirements tend to be considerably lower in first-episode patients, but some individuals may require higher doses than suggested. Studies in first-episode patients are not available with all drugs.*

	First Episode (mg)	Multiple episode (mg)
Clozapine*	100–200	400–900
Risperidone	2–4	4–10
Olanzapine	5–10	10–20
Quetiapine	200–400	400–750
Amisulpride	300–400	400–1200
Sertindole	8–10	12–20
Zotepine	100	100–300
Ziprasidone	40–60	40–160

*With the exception of Germany, Clozapine is not recommended unless patients have failed on other drugs.

cians believe that tardive dyskinesia is only a risk after years of chronic treatment, the incidence within the first year or two of treatment is similar to that seen in year four or five. With conventional antipsychotics the risk of tardive dyskinesia has been reported to be 5% even in the first year of treatment[67]. Since neurologic side-effects such as dystonia and akathisia can be extremely unpleasant and even frightening, the occurrence of these adverse effects can have unfortunate consequences in first-episode patients — creating a negative attitude toward medication and contributing to subsequent non-compliance. Although EPS can be prevented with the administration of concomitant antiparkinsonian drugs, these medications have their own side-effects and it is preferable to use antipsychotic drugs that are less likely to cause these reactions.

One of the major advantages of the new generation of 'atypical' antipsychotic drugs is their lower propensity to cause EPS, and emerging data support expectations that the risk of tardive dyskinesia would be substantially lower as well.[38,48,68] Most experts would argue that these advantages alone are sufficient to warrant the use of new-generation medications in the treatment of first-episode patients. Though the costs associated with the newer drugs may be higher the ultimate long-term advantages should support the cost-effectiveness of these medications.

In addition, the new-generation antipsychotic drugs have in some studies demonstrated superior efficacy against negative symptoms, depressive symptoms and cognitive dysfunction. These factors could contribute to enhanced quality of life, improved functional outcome and higher rates of compliance, as well as greater likelihood of participating in psychosocial and vocational therapies.

Antipsychotic drug dose

One question that has been raised about comparisons between new medications and conventional drugs is relative dose equivalence. In several studies dosages of haloperidol were used which some might argue were higher than necessary. Many of the studies with new medications used multiple doses of the new drug and only one dose of the comparator. An important study which addresses this concern was a seven-arm trial involving three dosages of haloperidol, three dosages of sertindole, and a placebo.[50] The lowest dose of haloperidol, 4 mg, was associated with significantly more EPS than any dose of sertindole or placebo. These data confirm that the advantages of the new drugs are not merely attributable to the dosage of the comparator (4 mg of haloperidol would be an effective dose in first-episode patients, but would generally be considered as too low for more chronic patients).

Most studies of first-episode patients have involved conventional antipsychotic medications. Data derived from clinical trials and PET studies suggest that low doses are effective in these patients.[69,70]

The overwhelming majority of first-episode patients respond well to treatment. In the Hillside first-episode study 83% of patients had achieved stable remission of psychotic signs and symptoms at the end of 1 year.[20] The median time to response was 11 weeks. For patients who fail to respond adequately, alternative treatments should be explored. Given the availability of several new-generation medications it is reasonable to try another of these drugs. It remains controversial whether adding or switching to a conventional drug increases the likelihood of responding in treatment-refractory patients. Clozapine should be tried in patients who have failed to respond to two or three other drugs (even when they have been new-generation medications).

In patients who are not responding adequately after several weeks of treatment there are a number of steps that should be taken. First, compliance should be checked by measuring blood levels which can help not only to confirm compliance, but also to identify individuals with unusually low blood levels despite adequate dosage. In such cases a strong rationale exists to initiate a trial of higher doses. There are a number of factors that can contribute to low blood levels (smoking, drug interactions, etc.).

The diagnosis should be reviewed in order to ensure that all available evidence supports the presumptive diagnosis of schizophrenia. Substance abuse should be considered, and ruled out. Evaluation of psychosocial stressors should be considered, and if they are identified further steps should be taken to reduce them and/or to help the patient cope with them. If an affective component is present the addition of a mood stabilizer or an antidepressant could be helpful (keep in mind that concomitant medications may alter the blood levels of the primary antipsychotic).

Many clinicians will increase dosage before switching to another antipsychotic drug. This is clearly indicated if blood levels are low, but its effectiveness beyond that has not been well established,[71] and more work needs to be done exploring higher dosage levels of the new-generation antipsychotic medications.

Deciding on how long to wait before switching to a different drug is also a challenge for clinicians and unfortunately there are no clinical trials to determine the optimum time to switch. As a general rule, some clinically significant improvement should be observed within the first 2 weeks and up to 50% of the ultimate improvement may be seen within 4 weeks. The problem remains, however, for patients who demonstrate definite improvement, but are left with more than minimal residual symptoms: is it worthwhile to try another medication, or is combination treatment appropriate? Although it is difficult to argue against a therapeutic trial, it is common to see patients who have been treated with multiple drugs without a clear indication of whether or not (and which ones) have been helpful. It is strongly recommended that first, the target symptoms and their level of severity should be documented, and second, that only one alteration in medication or dosage should be made at a time, so that a clear attribution can be made if improvement (or worsening) occurs. Often one of the most difficult challenges in reviewing patients' treatment histories is determining what impact specific treatments had. In addition, once a difficult patient is taking multiple medications there is a reluctance to discontinue any of them. It is important when making and documenting treatment decisions that clinicians take the perspective of someone who might be asked to take over the care of that patient in the future.

Continuation and maintenance treatment

The continuation phase is the period of treatment following recovery from an acute episode where stabilization and consolidation of therapeutic gains should be achieved. This can be a time of vulnerability to relapse or re-emergence of symptoms. The point at which continuation becomes maintenance or preventive treatment is not clear, but is generally thought to be 6–12 months.

There continues to be controversy as to what length of maintenance treatment is appropriate following recovery from a first episode. There are few controlled trials involving this specific population, but all of them demonstrate a significant reduction in the risk of relapse over 1–2 years in comparison with those patients receiving placebo.[72,73]

Current guidelines recommend maintenance treatment for 1–2 years following a first episode.[74,75] However, the follow-up studies of first-episode patients indicate that relapse rates of 80% after 5 years are to be expected (Table 10). If further deterioration of functional capacity occurs with each episode then we should extend recommendations toward longer intervals of maintenance treatment. The data from the Hillside prospective study indicated continued medication to be the single best predictor of continuing remission.[83]

Table 10 *Relapse following first episode of schizophrenia.*

Authors	Duration of follow-up (yr)	Percentage relapsed
Kane et al. (1982)[72]	3.5	69
Rabiner et al. (1986)[76]	1	29
Crow et al. (1986)[73]	2	55
Prudo and Blum (1987)[77]	5	80
McCreadie et al. (1988; 1992)[78,79]	5	70
Rajkumar and Thara (1989)[80]	3	59
Zhang et al. (1994)[81]	1.5	35
Linszen et al. (1994)[82]	1.5	17
Robinson et al. (1999)[83]	5	82

Extended periods of maintenance treatment for patients in remission require an ongoing assessment of risks and benefits as well as patient and family participation in this process. Many first-episode patients choose to discontinue medication within a year or two. It is also clear that not all patients experience a relapse (even over a 5-year follow-up period). Unfortunately, there are no good predictors of which patients can sustain remission in a drug-free state.

The possibility of targeted or intermittent treatment has been suggested as an alternative to continuous medication. For multiple-episode patients this approach has been disappointing, but for first-episode patients who do not wish to continue taking medication this strategy may provide the best hope of early intervention if and when a relapse does occur. A recurrent problem, however, is that many first-episode patients will not even agree to regular clinical follow-up after medication is discontinued.

The dosage in maintenance treatment should be as low as possible. Some dosage guidelines exist for the conventional drugs, but these data were generally obtained from studies involving multiple-episode patients. The findings that first-episode patients can respond to relatively low doses during acute treatment suggest the need for low maintenance dosages.

The use of depot drugs should be considered, as this can enhance compliance, or at least make non-compliance obvious. However, at present none of the new-generation medications is available in a long-acting preparation, so the choice becomes somewhat more complicated.

Treatment of subsequent episodes

The management of acute relapse or exacerbations in patients who have already had at least one episode requires a different approach in terms of evaluation and treatment planning compared with patients presenting with a first episode.

At this stage of the illness more information is available to confirm or support a diagnosis which previously might have been presumptive. Symptom patterns and chronology should be re-evaluated and further documented. A critical question is what — if any — precipitating factors were involved in leading to a relapse, and how such factors will influence the treatment plan. Specifically, did the patient relapse after discontinuing medication, or did the relapse occur despite continued antipsychotic medication (with evidence of compliance)? In some cases the sequence of events can be unclear. An antipsychotic drug blood level could be helpful in determining whether medication is still present, although this would only provide a qualitative rather than quantitative estimate of the degree of compliance. Other factors such as substance abuse or stressful life events should also be considered. If a possibility of substance abuse exists, urine screening could be helpful in clarifying this issue. The potential reasons for relapse should be investigated and documented as rapidly as possible, since with the passage of time tests such as drug urine screens and antipsychotic drug blood levels may become less meaningful.

Determining whether or not a relapse has occurred despite maintenance medication could have implications for both acute and long-term treatment strategies, and a documentation of non-compliance would be important in informing subsequent relapse prevention strategies.

The choice of drug and dosage will also be influenced by an evaluation of past treatment response. If a patient has a history of responding well to a particular agent, that medication should be considered a first choice unless other factors (adverse effects, non-compliance) come into play. If a patient has relapsed despite adequate dosage and compliance a re-evaluation of that medication choice and dosage should take place. Many clinicians assume that if a relapse has occurred on a specific dose then an increase in dose would be an appropriate management strategy. It is not clear, however, whether switching to another drug or increasing the dose is the more useful strategy, and in fact one study suggested that improvement occurred with hospitalization and no change in dosage.[84]

If the patient has been on a conventional agent and there is reason to switch, a new-generation antipsychotic should be considered. One situation that would currently support the use of conventional agents would be if a long-acting preparation is indicated. At present it is a difficult choice given the lack of availability of long-acting forms of new-generation medications. Although there is reason to be optimistic that the newer drugs will be associated with better compliance, there is no systematic long-term study of this issue and no controlled comparison of depot drugs versus new-generation medications.

The dosage required to treat a second or subsequent episode might be somewhat higher than that required to treat a first episode, but there are no longitudinal data establishing minimum effective dose from one episode to the next, and we have little knowledge as to when and why dosage requirements change over time. There can be some degree of enzyme induction over time with antipsychotic drugs, but good estimates are lacking.

Treatment should initially focus on bringing acute symptoms under control and establishing a long-range treatment plan. If acute symptoms do not respond adequately clinicians face difficult decisions as to when and how to alter the initial treatment (see Managing the poor or partial responder).

Different clinical situations will influence the rapidity with which initial medication and dosage are altered. Some degree of response is expected within the first 1–2 weeks, though the ultimate degree of response can take considerably longer. The severity of symptoms and the treatment environment can also influence the time clinicians can wait for an initial response. If a reasonable degree of improvement is observed, the next step is the management of adverse effects, initiation of appropriate psychosocial and rehabilitative services, and planning and implementation of patient and family psychoeducation. In many health-care systems there is pressure to reduce length of hospital stays and the more careful planning that can be done prior to discharge the more likely it is that successful follow-up care can be implemented.

Management of adverse effects

Extrapyramidal side-effects

Extrapyramidal side-effects (EPS) are particularly important because with conventional antipsychotic drugs they are common, potentially distressing, often misdiagnosed, and can lead to functional impairment and non-compliance. One of the major advantages of new-generation drugs is a substantially reduced propensity to cause these effects. When these reactions do occur they can be treated with antiparkinsonian medication or a reduction in dosage. The occurrence of an acute dystonic reaction should be treated with intramuscular medication, either anticholinergic or antihistaminic. A beta-blocker such as propranolol may be helpful in treating akathisia. Benzodiazepines can also be helpful. It can be difficult at times to differentiate akathisia from anxiety or psychotic agitation.

Tardive dyskinesia

The problem of abnormal involuntary movements associated with long-term exposure to conventional antipsychotic agents has been one of the most serious concerns regarding their use. At the same time it is clear from an extensive series of studies that long-term treatment has enormous advantages in terms of preventing psychotic relapse and rehospitalization and maintaining optimum levels of adjustment in the community.

With conventional antipsychotic medication the cumulative incidence of tardive dyskinesia is approximately 5% per year.[85] Even during the first year of neuroleptic exposure to these drugs the risk is as high as 5%. In older patients the risk can be 25–30% within 1 year.[86] Though cases of tardive dyskinesia have been reported with the new-generation drugs, in systematic follow-up studies or controlled trials the incidence appears to be significantly lower than with conventional agents.

Many would argue that this factor alone is sufficient to justify the choice of new over old medications. Though most cases of tardive dyskinesia are mild, some can be persistent and severe. Even mild cases can add to the stigma associated with schizophrenia, as even subtle abnormal movements contribute to patients looking 'peculiar'. There is no proven safe and effective treatment for tardive dyskinesia; therefore drug discontinuation or switching to a different medication are the preferred initial strategies.

Sedation

Sedation is a common effect of antipsychotic therapy. At times (during acute treatment of agitation) this can be a desirable effect. Later on in treatment it can be highly undesirable. Giving medication all or largely at night can be helpful. Dose reduction or changing to a less sedating medication are alternative strategies.

Weight gain

Substantial increase in weight is one of the more troublesome side-effects of new-generation medications.

Figure 2 provides a comparison of amount of weight gain after 10 weeks of treatment with a variety of medications. Clozapine and olanzapine are generally associated with the greatest degree of weight gain. Although some have suggested that weight gain was a positive sign in that it was associated with good clinical response, this has not been the author's experience.[87] Although weight gain is troubling in the short term and can lead to non-

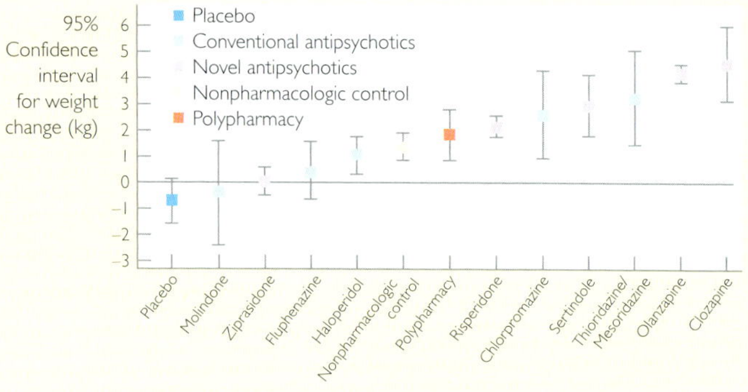

Figure 2 *95% confidence intervals for weight change after 10 weeks on standard drug doses, estimated from a random effects model. Reprinted with permission from Allison et al.*[18]

compliance, there is also considerable concern about the long-term health consequences. Concern has also been raised regarding the development of impaired glucose tolerance and the development of diabetes mellitus. Abnormal glucose tolerance has been reported in 10% of clozapine-treated patients.[88] These effects do not seem to be merely a consequence of weight increase. Patients with pre-existing diabetes or with known risk factors should have assessment of glucose tolerance prior to and during antipsychotic drug treatment.

Although dietary control and exercise are important, it may be necessary to switch medications to one that has less effect on weight gain. Some clinicians use adjunctive pharmacologic treatments (e.g. methylphenidate, sibutramine, topiramate), but long-term data in this context are lacking.

Endocrine effects

Hyperprolactinaemia has been associated with conventional antipsychotic drugs. New-generation medications tend to have much less effect on prolactin, with risperidone being the most likely and quetiapine and clozapine the least likely to cause prolactin elevation. Hyperprolactinaemia is reversible upon stopping medication. It can be associated with painful or swollen breasts, galactorrhoea, amenorrhoea and sexual dysfunction, but in general the relationship between prolactin levels and these potential side-effects is not consistently apparent.

Sexual dysfunction

Erectile dysfunction is commonly seen in patients taking antipsychotic medication, but this and other sexual side-effects have received inadequate attention. Ejaculatory disturbances (including occasionally retrograde ejaculation) and loss of libido can occur in men, and diminished libido and anorgasmia can occur in women. Reducing dosage or switching medications is sometimes necessary. Imipramine has been used for treating retrograde ejaculation. Yohimbine or cyproheptadine has been helpful for some patients with erectile dysfunction, as has sildenafil.

Seizures

Many antipsychotic drugs, particularly the low-potency conventional antipsychotics and clozapine, can lower the seizure threshold. In the case of clozapine there is debate as to to what extent this phenomenon is dose-related, but some reports suggest an incidence above 10% among patients receiving high doses. When a seizure does occur the dose should be reduced and a neurologic evaluation conducted. If clozapine has proved to be helpful it can in most cases be continued. Valproate would be the preferred anticonvulsant given the risk of agranulocytosis associated with carbamazepine.

Autonomic effects

Drugs with strong anticholinergic properties can produce dry mouth, blurred vision, constipation, tachycardia, urinary retention and impaired cognitive functioning. In general these effects are not prominent with new-generation antipsychotics. These effects can be particularly troubling in the elderly. Prolongation of the QT_c interval has received increasing attention as a risk factor for ventricular fibrillation, particularly torsade des pointes, and has led to limitations on the use of some medications (e.g. sertindole). Controversy remains as to the threshold of risk associated with slight increases in the QT_c interval.

Orthostatic hypotension occurs to varying degrees with antipsychotic drugs depending upon adrenergic antagonist properties. Gradual dosage escalation can be helpful. Patients should be instructed to rise slowly from a seated or prone position. At times switching to another medication is necessary.

Haematological effects

Leukopenia occurs in a proportion (5–10%) of patients receiving antipsychotic medications. Usually this is a benign reaction, but agranulocytosis can occur with conventional drugs. It is the most serious risk associated with clozapine treatment and occurs in 0.4–1.0% of patients. With early detection and appropriate management fatal outcomes are extremely rare. To date, there have been no reported cases of agranulocytosis attributable to any other of the new-generation medications.

Hepatic effects

Abnormalities in liver transaminases have been observed with typical antipsychotic agents, and occasionally cholestatic jaundice occurs. The latter is much less frequent than in the early days of neuroleptic treatment, for reasons that are not entirely clear.

Liver function test abnormalities are reported in approximately 1% of patients receiving new-generation medications. They are usually transient and rarely result in the need to discontinue the medication. However, patients with hepatic disease may require increased consideration and surveillance.

Skin and eye effects

Dermatologic allergic reactions including maculopapular rash, swelling and urticaria can occur with antipsychotic agents. Chlorpromazine in particular has been associated with phototoxic skin reactions. Doses of thioridazine in excess of 800 mg/day are contraindicated because of concerns regarding pigmentary retinopathy.

In one species of dog which is known to be particularly susceptible to the development of cataracts, but not in monkeys, quetiapine was associated with lens opacity and cataracts. To date, despite widespread use of the drug, there has been no clinical evidence of any problem.

Neuroleptic malignant syndrome

Neuroleptic malignant syndrome (NMS) is a potentially fatal but rare adverse effect of antipsychotic medication. The incidence appears to be significantly lower with new-generation antipsychotics, although rare cases have been reported with clozapine and risperidone (often in the context of co-administration of other psychotropic drugs). Although controlled trials are not available because of the nature and severity of the condition, bromocriptine and dantrolene are the standard treatments along with discontinuation of the antipsychotic and appropriate medical management.

The adverse effects of new-generation medications are summarized in Table 11.

Table 11 *Adverse effects of new-generation antipsychotic drugs.*

Clozapine	Orthostatic hypotension, sedation, tachycardia, weight gain, hypersalivation, seizures Agranulocytosis occurs in 0.5–0.8% of patients
Risperidone	Insomnia, nausea, agitation, EPS (at high doses), fatigue, orthostatic dizziness, weight gain
Olanzapine	Somnolence, constipation, weight gain, dry mouth, dizziness
Quetiapine	Somnolence, headache, dizziness
Amisulpride	Insomnia, anxiety, agitation, constipation, nausea, dry mouth
Sertindole	Headache, rhinitis, dizziness, QT_C prolongation, diminished ejaculatory volume

Managing the poor or partial responder

Poor or partial response implies that despite seemingly adequate pharmacologic treatment symptoms persist which are considered to be a problem. Usually positive symptoms are the focus of these concerns, but severe affective symptoms, cognitive dysfunction, anxiety or negative symptoms can also be significant aspects of defining response. Definitions of poor or partial response vary, but most would agree that failure to respond adequately to two different drugs given in adequate doses for 4–6 weeks each would be part of the definition.

When poor response occurs a number of steps should precede altering the treatment plan. The diagnosis should be reviewed, co-morbid conditions (e.g. substance abuse) should be reconsidered and compliance and potentially idiosyncratic drug metabolism should be evaluated. Once these factors have been considered clinicians are faced with a number of alternatives: waiting in the hope that the patient is just slow to respond, increasing the dose, adding adjunctive pharmacologic treatment, or switching to a different antipsychotic agent.

High-dose treatment

Most of the studies involving high or 'mega' doses have failed to demonstrate significant improvement.[89,90] There are few data available for the new-generation drugs comparing conventional doses with high-dose treatment in poor or partial responders.

Switching medication

Switching to another class of drug has been studied infrequently in a systematic controlled fashion, since improvement following a change in drug could be due to passage of time. Controlled comparisons of patients who undergo a change and patients who stay on the original treatment are necessary to address this issue. For example, Kinon et al. studied a sample of 156 acutely ill patients with schizophrenia who were treated openly for 4 weeks with fluphenazine 20 mg/day.[71] Patients who had residual psychotic signs and symptoms at the end of the 4-week trial were then randomly assigned, double blind, to one of three treatments: (1) continued fluphenazine 20 mg/day; (2) fluphenazine 80 mg/day; or (3) haloperidol 20 mg/day. This second treatment phase lasted an additional 4 weeks. Fifty-eight patients were eligible and agreed to participate in the second part of the study and 47 provided analysable data. Only four patients (9%) achieved a good clinical response during the controlled comparison and no significant differences between the treatments were evident. These results suggest that for patients who did not respond at 4 weeks, the alternative treatment strategies applied over the next 4 weeks did not bring about substantial further response.

The possibility that a longer trial of an alternative treatment could have brought about further improvement cannot be ruled out. In addition, this trial involved switching from one conventional agent to another. The possibility that the new-generation medications would be more effective in this context also requires study.

Clozapine

Among the new-generation antipsychotic medications, clozapine has provided the most compelling and consistent evidence for effectiveness in patients who have been poor or partial responders to conventional drugs. There are a number of controlled trials that demonstrate clozapine's superiority, particularly in reducing positive symptoms,[23] but also in reducing rates of relapse and rehospitalization in chronic refractory patients.[91,92] It is also clear that not all patients respond to clozapine, and a persistent concern is how to manage patients who do not benefit from this treatment.

The first question in such cases would be the adequacy of the clozapine treatment trial, both in terms of dosage and duration. Several studies have reported that plasma levels above a threshold of 350–400 ng/ml are associated with the highest likelihood of response.[93–95] The duration of an adequate trial is more debatable, but most would agree that a trial of clozapine of 3–6 months should achieve some clinically significant improvement in psychopathology. This by no means implies that all of the potential improvement would be seen within that interval; but some meaningful improvement should occur.

Clearly, because of clozapine's risk of producing agranulocytosis, weekly blood monitoring is necessary (at least during the early phase of treatment). Unfortunately, apart from plasma levels there is no well-established predictor of clozapine response; therefore a therapeutic trial is warranted for patients who have failed to respond to other drugs.

With the introduction of other 'atypical' or new-generation drugs modelled to varying degrees on clozapine, the logical question arises as to their effectiveness in poorly or partially responsive patients. There are studies with risperidone, olanzapine and quetiapine[49] suggesting that some proportion of such patients will benefit;[33,43] however, the data are not as extensive as those involving clozapine. At the same time, since these drugs are easier to administer, it is logical to initiate a therapeutic trial of one (or possibly two) of them before turning to clozapine. We do not have data yet to guide us as to whether one or two trials of a new-generation drug are appropriate before switching to clozapine, but a trial of clozapine is definitely appropriate in patients who have inadequate responses to other new-generation drugs.

Augmentation with other antipsychotic drugs

A number of studies have examined the potential benefit of adding another antipsychotic agent to an ineffective drug regimen. In the case of clozapine augmentation some efficacy has been demonstrated with pimozide,[96] risperidone,[97] sulpiride,[98] and loxapine.[99]

Although many clinicians are combining first- and second-generation medications in the management of poor or partial responders, there are as yet insufficient data to support the value of these combinations. Switching to a second-generation medication is recommended rather than adding it to a conventional drug.

Other adjunctive treatments

An additional possibility is the use of other classes of psychotropic medication as adjuncts to antipsychotics. Lithium and other mood stabilizers, benzodiazepines and antidepressants have been used in this context.

Lithium has been reported to be helpful in a number of double-blind trials.[100–102] However, other studies did not confirm this effect.[103,104] Schulz et al. have reported on the largest sample of poor or partially responsive patients with schizophrenia randomly assigned to antipsychotic plus lithium or antipsychotic plus placebo. This trial did not demonstrate any significant advantage for adjunctive lithium.[105]

Anticonvulsants such as carbamazepine and sodium valproate have also been added to antipsychotics. Carbamazepine has been the most widely studied. Out of nine treatment trials reviewed by Schulz et al. four included patients specifically identified as violent or aggressive.[106] Patients with excitement, impulsivity and aggressive behaviour as well as those showing non-specific electroencephalographic abnormalities may be more likely to experience improvement with anticonvulsants. The extent to which these symptom patterns represent manic behaviour is also an important consideration. Valproate has also been helpful in such patients. Adverse effects of these drugs should be taken into consideration. Carbamazepine is a potent inducer of hepatic enzymes and concomitant administration can cause a 50% or greater reduction in blood levels of antipsychotic medication.[107]

Benzodiazepines have also been used as adjunctive treatment. Often this is to control acute agitation during the early phase of treatment as antipsychotic drugs are being initiated, but these agents have also been used in an attempt to enhance response in refractory patients. Although some studies suggest a positive effect,[108] others do not,[109] and there does not appear to be a specific antipsychotic effect.[110]

Antidepressants have been widely used as adjunctive treatments, but primarily to treat co-morbid depression or 'post-psychotic' depression.[111] There is no evidence that they are helpful in treating refractory positive symptoms. Antidepressants can improve negative symptoms,[112] but maximum benefit can take as long as 12 weeks. Siris et al. conducted a placebo-controlled continuation trial of 24 schizophrenic or schizoaffective patients with post-psychotic depression who had initially proved responsive to the antidepressant. During the subsequent 1-year follow-up, patients receiving placebo were not only more likely to suffer a recurrence of a depressive episode, but were also more likely to suffer a psychotic relapse.[111] This is an intriguing finding, but unfortunately it has not been further explored. These findings also raise important questions about potential overlap between depressive and negative symptoms and the potential role of depression in psychotic relapse.

In using antidepressants in conjunction with antipsychotic agents it is important to be aware of potential pharmacokinetic interactions. Drugs that inhibit liver enzymes involved in metabolizing specific drugs could lead to clinically significant and potentially toxic increases in drug blood levels.

Electroconvulsive therapy (ECT) is another adjunctive treatment which has been shown to be helpful. It has been suggested that the effects of ECT and antipsychotic medications can be synergistic.[113] Several reports of small case series have indicated that ECT can be effective as an adjunct to clozapine in treatment-refractory patients.[114,115] Chanpattana et al. reported on 114 treatment-resistant patients who were treated with ECT and flupenthixol 12–24 mg/day: 58 per cent showed significant improvement, and when ECT was discontinued the rate of relapse was significantly higher than among those who continued to receive the combined treatment for an additional 6 months.[116] This underscores the potentially time-limited effects of ECT in this context; however, maintenance ECT can be given at less frequent intervals and may be sufficient to sustain the improvement.

The data on alternative adjunctive treatments suggest that none is consistently effective and none is superior or even equivalent to clozapine. In addition, given emerging data that some refractory patients can benefit from other new-generation drugs (risperidone and olanzapine are the most widely studied) it makes sense to try these agents first. A critical factor in initiating a therapeutic trial of any of these agents is to document the target symptoms and their response over time to the new treatment in such a way that a determination can be made as to its effectiveness. In addition, if possible, only one new treatment (or significant change in dosage) should be implemented at a time so that a reasonable attribution of cause and effect can be made. All too often it is difficult to evaluate the impact of these treatment approaches, and many patients continue to receive multiple drugs for long periods when it is not clear what benefits have accrued.

Long-term therapeutic management

Soon after the introduction of antipsychotic medications studies were initiated not only to determine their impact in the control of acute signs and symptoms, but also their potential role in preventing subsequent exacerbations or relapse. A number of placebo-controlled trials documented the efficacy of continued medication.[117–119] Overall relapse rates on placebo averaged 70–75%, whereas relapse rates on active medication were only 20–25%. Initially, far fewer data were collected on other aspects of the disease such as psychosocial, vocational and cognitive functioning.

Shortly after the long-term use of antipsychotic medication became clinically justified, increasing concern developed regarding the potential long-term adverse effects associated with these drugs. Although tardive dyskinesia was first described shortly after the introduction of antipsychotic medication, considerable debate and uncertainty remained about its prevalence, incidence, severity and even its relationship to drug exposure.[120]

Following further investigation and the introduction of prospective designs it became increasingly apparent that the association between exposure to first-generation antipsychotic medication and tardive dyskinesia was real (though some cases can occur without drug exposure) and that the incidence was approximately 5% per year of drug exposure with relatively consistent risk occurring for the first 8–10 years of treatment.[121] In elderly patients treated with conventional antipsychotic drugs the risk has been shown to be approximately five times higher.[86,122,123] In addition, a number of studies have suggested a relationship between early parkinsonism and later tardive dyskinesia.[86]

The introduction of the new-generation antipsychotic drugs provides an important advantage in reducing the risk of tardive dyskinesia and enhancing the benefit-to-risk ratio of long-term maintenance treatment.

Compliance

Compliance in medication-taking is a considerable problem in any chronic disease. In a condition such as schizophrenia the challenge is even greater because the disease itself can interfere with insight, judgment and motivation. In addition, considerable stigma is associated with the illness and many health systems remain fragmented and badly integrated when dealing with the chronically mentally ill. Factors contributing to non-compliance are outlined in Table 12.

Long-acting, depot medications can be helpful in reducing rates of non-compliance, or at least making it obvious when non-compliance does occur.[124] On the other hand, patients may refuse to take injections, and as yet there are no long-acting formulations

Table 12 *Factors contributing to non-compliance in schizophrenia.*

Patient-related factors	Lack of adequate information Symptom severity Lack of insight Denial Co-morbid conditions (e.g. substance abuse)
Treatment-related factors	Medication side-effects Inadequate therapeutic alliance Inconvenient regimen
Environmental factors	Inadequate social support Insufficient funds or access

of the new-generation antipsychotic medications. It is hoped that their better safety and tolerability profile will improve compliance rates, but a number of other factors also influence compliance.

For example, a randomized, controlled trial of compliance therapy found an impact on post-treatment measures of insight, attitudes to treatment and observer-rated compliance.[125] Survival in the community prior to readmission was significantly longer in the compliance therapy group. The compliance therapy provided consisted of four to six sessions based on motivational interviewing, cognitive psychoeducational approaches to psychotic symptoms and underscoring the importance of the treatment alliance and patient participation.

Although the study involved a relatively small sample and requires replication it adds to a large body of data stressing the importance of a number of non-pharmacologic treatment strategies in enhancing long-term outcome. This is particularly important since reviews of the literature on medication adherence in schizophrenia suggest that insight and health beliefs are important determinants of compliance, as are available social support, substance abuse co-morbidity and the quality of the therapeutic alliance.[126] A number of strategies to enhance compliance are listed in Table 13.

In the Hillside Hospital first episode study, Robinson et al. examined the characteristics of patients who had recovered from their first episode, subsequently stopped taking medication, relapsed, responded a second time to treatment, but then became non-compliant.[127] Compared with patients who continued to take medication, those who stopped had better premorbid adjustment, a later onset of psychotic symptoms and better neurocognitive performance. These data suggest that patients who have better functioning are more likely to deny that they have an ongoing illness. It is possible that this relationship may change over time as more relapses occur. These findings under-

Table 13 *General interventions to maximize the likelihood of compliance. From Fenton et al.*[126]

- Conduct an assessment of compliance history and risk factors, including substance abuse and financial or other practical barriers, as part of the evaluation of every patient
- Allow sufficient time to know the patient as a person and to understand his or her personal goals, concerns, and psychodynamic issues. Place assisting the patient in meeting self-defined goals at the centre of treatment
- Use a negotiated approach to medication. Create a therapeutic environment where deviation from recommendations can be discussed openly, rather than concealed. Show an interest in medication by asking in a non-authoritarian manner how much is being taken and the effects. Involve the patient in medication treatment by allowing self-regulation of dosage, if possible
- Maximize efficacy and minimize side-effects in choosing agents and dosages. Attend seriously to all side-effects and actively elicit and respond to concerns
- Educate patient and family regarding the biological underpinnings of illness, relapse prevention and medication side-effects
- Enlist support in the community, including family, friends and employers. If needed, arrange for supervised medication administration
- Employ cognitive and memory-enhancing strategies if disorganization or forgetfulness is a problem
- When the patient is rendered incompetent because of illness, be prepared to recommend judicial intervention
- If the patient will not comply and is competent, manage counter transference to allow for a continued relationship and the possibility of future treatment

score the importance of psychoeducation in meeting the challenges of long-term compliance.

Indications for maintenance treatment

In recent years a number of guidelines have been published regarding indications for maintenance treatment.[74,75,128] Following recovery from a first episode of psychosis associated with a schizophrenic illness, 1–2 years is usually the recommendation. After two or more episodes, 5 years or longer is the usual suggestion. Although it is rare to see recommendations suggesting indefinite long-term treatment, the available evidence would suggest that to be a reasonable recommendation.

To a large extent these recommendations have been influenced not only by potential benefits, but also by the risks associated with the long-term use of conventional antipsychotics. As the new generation of medications are demonstrated to be associated with a significantly reduced risk of adverse effects such as tardive dyskinesia, then modifications in the long-term treatment recommendations should be considered. (Unfortunately, as is the case in many medical specialties, controlled trials are not always available to inform everyday decisions in clinical practice. There are numerous trials lasting 1–2 years in the maintenance treatment of schizophrenia, but few trials have lasted for longer periods and we, therefore, must rely on naturalistic follow-up data to estimate the risk of relapse over longer periods of time.)

A particularly challenging situation for clinicians and patients occurs when an individual has been in relatively good remission for a long period and questions arise as to whether the medication continues to be necessary. It is not surprising that when an individual has been well for a long time a sense of security or invulnerability may develop. Though few controlled trials involving random assignment have been done, there are a number of naturalistic follow-up studies of individuals who had been in good remission for as long as 5 years prior to discontinuing medication.[129] The mean relapse rate among such individuals over the next 1–2 years was shown to approximate 75%. These findings suggest caution in discontinuing medication even in patients who have been in good remission for long periods. It might also be argued that given the gains that these patients have made, they have an enormous amount to lose if and when a psychotic relapse does occur.

Another clinical situation about which there is uncertainty, hesitancy and reluctance on the part of patients is following recovery from the very first psychotic episode in a schizophrenic illness. Again, unfortunately, there are very few controlled, random-assignment, clinical trials of maintenance treatment following recovery from a first episode. Those that have been conducted are consistent in demonstrating a significant effect of medication in reducing the risk of relapse over 1–2 years following recovery.[73,130] It is also clear, however, that not all patients in this context will experience a relapse within the first year or two, even if medication is discontinued. Data available from longer-term naturalistic follow-up studies suggest that the relapse rate among first-episode patients is at least 75% over the subsequent 5 years. For example, Robinson et al. reported relapse data from the Hillside Hospital first episode study: 104 patients responded to the treatment of their index episode; 5 years after recovery from their previous episode, the cumulative rate of first relapse in patients who were at risk was 82%; the rate for a second relapse was 78%.[127] Survival analysis showed that not taking antipsychotic medication increased the risk of relapse by almost five times.[83] Subsequent analysis controlling for antipsychotic usage showed that patients with poor premorbid adaptation to school and premorbid social withdrawal relapsed earlier (these data may suggest that patients with more obvious neurodevelopmental aspects to the illness might have a greater vulnerability to early relapse).

The consequences of relapse in individuals during this phase of illness can be dramatic, particularly since first-episode patients usually do achieve a good remission of psychotic signs and symptoms and have a reasonable chance of returning to work or school. Subsequent relapses, therefore, can be associated with significant declines in psychosocial and vocational adjustment and possibly less robust symptomatic improvement.

Existing guidelines do not strongly recommend treatment beyond 1–2 years in first-episode patients, and even in multi-episode patients these recommendations do not generally exceed 5 years. There is no evidence that the risk of relapse declines substantially after 5 years in multi-episode patients. Reports including patients in good remission for long periods still find an average relapse rate of 75% within 1–2 years of discontinuation of medication.

With the observed variability in time course of relapse and concomitant concerns over continuous treatment with medications that might have side-effects, numerous analyses have been carried out to identify predictors of relapse, ranging from clinical measures, symptom patterns and severity, to historical measures such as length of illness and patient variables such as age, sex or diagnostic subtype. In addition, biological variables such as brain morphology, neurotransmitter levels or responsivity to pharmacologic challenges have also been studied. The overall conclusion is that no predictors of outcome demonstrate sufficient predictive power and feasibility to apply on a routine clinical basis. Clearly, the continuation of medication is the most powerful intervention for the prevention of relapse. One variable that has not been studied systematically is the rapidity with which medication is discontinued. Relapse may occur significantly sooner (though not immediately) in patients who rapidly discontinue all medication in comparison with those who discontinue gradually or those who discontinue depot medication.[131] This is a clinical point to keep in mind when patients are discontinuing their medication for whatever reason.

New-generation antipsychotic drugs and maintenance treatment

The introduction of new-generation antipsychotic medications will facilitate the effectiveness of maintenance treatment in a number of ways. First, the concern regarding tardive dyskinesia should diminish. The newer drugs have a significantly reduced risk of extrapyramidal side-effects, and preliminary results suggest a lower incidence of tardive dyskinesia as well.[68,132,133] In addition, the newer drugs may be better tolerated in a variety of other respects. However, weight gain is a current concern and the focus of additional research and preventive strategies. Indications that the new-generation drugs may also improve some aspects of cognitive functioning are promising and could have important functional implications (though this remains to be fully established). Further improvement in negative symptoms can have important functional consequences.

It is also clear that despite adequate maintenance treatment (even with guaranteed medication delivery) a substantial proportion of patients will relapse. Estimates from available studies suggest that approximately 20% of patients will relapse during the course of a year even with adequate pharmacologic treatment. When potential non-compliance is an additional factor then as many as 40–50% of patients may experience a relapse within a year. There are two major questions which need to be addressed regarding new-generation medications. First, can they succeed in preventing the 'breakthroughs' or the loss of effectiveness in a substantial number of patients receiving conventional medications? Second, will the newer drugs be associated with a greater degree of long-term compliance in medication-taking?

The management of negative symptoms

The management of negative symptoms

Increasing attention has been focused on negative symptoms as both a target of treatment and a clue to underlying pathophysiology. The treatment implications are enormous, because negative symptoms can persist despite treatment with conventional (and even new) antipsychotic medications and contribute substantially to the psychosocial and vocational disability associated with this illness. Negative symptoms are not merely a result of chronicity; they can be present during the early acute phase of the illness and as prodromal symptoms before the onset of florid positive symptoms. Presence of negative symptoms, particularly severe negative symptoms, at the onset of the illness has been associated with a poor outcome, although it is important to recognize that some aspects of functional impairment are included in the definition of negative symptoms in most classifications.

Differential diagnosis

In evaluating and planning treatment strategies for negative symptoms it is important to consider potential confounds. Some have attempted to divide negative symptoms into primary and secondary, while others have used the 'deficit state' concept to categorize patients in whom other potential causes of negative symptoms have been ruled out (at least to the extent possible).[6] Phenomena that can mimic negative symptoms are depression, demoralization, antipsychotic drug-induced parkinsonian side-effects, withdrawal in response to frightening delusions or hallucinations, or the effects of chronic institutionalization. Eliminating these potential confounds is not necessarily a simple task.[6] For example, in one study of antipsychotic drug-naive, first-episode patients, 17% were found to have what appeared to be extrapyramidal signs similar to drug-induced parkinsonism, suggesting a pre-existing dysfunction in a proportion of patients.[134] These individuals were found to have more negative symptoms and to be more vulnerable to drug-induced EPS when they did ultimately receive antipsychotic medications. This suggests that extrapyramidal function is involved in the disease process, possibly related to negative symptoms, and not merely an adverse effect of antipsychotic drugs. Another concern is the length of time for which drug-induced parkinsonian side-effects can persist after drug withdrawal (in some cases weeks rather than days). This complicates the assessment of treatment effects when patients are switched from a conventional antipsychotic agent to a new-generation medication and only short-term impact on negative symptoms is examined.

New antipsychotic medications

The new-generation antipsychotic medications are associated in some studies with greater improvement in measures of negative symptoms than conventional drugs.[38,45,50,135,136] Even if this superiority is to some extent attributable to a lower burden of EPS, the ultimate benefit to the patient is important. Some studies have used statistical techniques such as path analysis to assess the impact of drug treatment on negative symptoms that is independent of improvement in positive symptoms and/or EPS.[137] The critical issues are whether long-term improvement in negative symptoms can be demonstrated and whether the functional impairment attributable to negative symptoms can ultimately be diminished.

Other medication strategies

A number of other classes of medication have been explored as treatments (usually adjunctive to antipsychotics) for negative symptoms. Antidepressants have been shown to have some beneficial effect in patients treated for co-morbid depression.[112,138] It is important to recognize that a number of features of depression and negative symptoms overlap. Anergia, anhedonia, reduced appetitive drives and inattention can be seen in both conditions. Yet some features may distinguish these conditions. Patients with depression usually describe a state of feeling 'blue' or 'down', but this is not the case in patients with negative symptoms. True flat affect is seen in individuals with negative symptoms, but not in the case of depression.

Recent interest in potential dysfunction of excitatory amino acids neurotransmission in schizophrenia has led to the development of treatment strategies based on this model. Some reports suggest that high-dose glycine or the antituberculosis drug D-cycloserine may be helpful in improving negative symptoms in some patients.[139,140] Further work is necessary to establish the value of this approach.

The evaluation and management of cognitive dysfunction

It has long been appreciated that schizophrenia is associated with a variety of cognitive impairments; however, in recent years attention has focused on developing specific therapeutic strategies to target this domain. The pathophysiology of cognitive dysfunction is far from clear and to some extent these abnormalities may represent the sequelae of neurodevelopmental abnormalities. This notion is supported by 'follow back' studies suggesting evidence of cognitive problems long before the onset of the disease, and the fact that cognitive impairments are present before the onset of psychosis.

Cognitive performance has been shown to be a predictor of functional outcome in schizophrenia,[141] and contributes enormously to psychosocial and vocational disability. While conventional antipsychotic drugs have demonstrated dramatic effects in alleviating positive symptoms and reducing the risk of psychotic relapse, they have not demonstrated consistent significant therapeutic effects on cognitive functioning. In fact, because antiparkinsonian, anticholinergic medications are frequently required to prevent or treat parkinsonian side-effects, the net effect of this combination is sometimes further decrement in memory performance. In addition, it is possible that a tendency to use higher than necessary doses of conventional antipsychotics contributed to minimal improvement in cognitive function and that lower doses could be more effective in this context.[142]

Advances in neuropsychology have also helped to develop a broader array of relevant tests. Preliminary evidence with new-generation antipsychotic medications is promising in suggesting that these agents can improve cognitive functioning to a measurable and statistically significant extent.[143,144] It remains to be seen whether these effects will result in meaningful changes in long-term functional outcome.

Assessing cognitive impairment

Patients with schizophrenia generally have levels of performance on cognitive tests which are 1–3 standard deviations below the norm based on their age and educational level.[145] This would mean that the typical patient with schizophrenia is in the bottom 15% of the population in cognitive performance. On measures of intelligence quotient, patients with schizophrenia generally score only 10 points below normative standards.[146] This suggests that intellectual functioning is reasonably well preserved in contrast to specific domains such as memory, attention and executive function. The cognitive impairments in schizophrenia appear to be relatively stable over time even when patients are assessed during a psychotic episode and again after improvement in positive symptoms. Cognitive dysfunction is, to some extent, correlated with severity of negative symptoms.[147]

Specific cognitive deficits have implications for particular domains of real-life functioning and an awareness of these limitations should help inform rehabilitative and pharmacologic approaches. Individuals who have difficulty with attention or vigilance may not be able to learn adequate social skills and may perform poorly in social situations. Problems with executive function can be associated with poor job performance, and memory deficits can impede the learning of new skills. It may be that insight into one's illness and ability to comply with medication on a regular basis are also associated with aspects of cognitive dysfunction.

For the average clinician assessment of cognitive function is usually not included in routine evaluations. A mental status examination as usually conducted is insufficient to identify specific abnormalities. Standardized tests to assess learning, memory, attention and executive function can be administered by a neuropsychologist or psychometrician during an initial assessment. A reasonable battery could be completed in an hour.

The role of new-generation drugs

A number of open-label and double-blind trials have been conducted with new-generation antipsychotic medications.[143,144,148] The results are encouraging, but not all studies report the same effects, even with specific drugs. Clozapine has been associated with improvements in executive function, verbal fluency and fine motor function, and risperidone has been associated with improvement in attention and executive function. Positive results have also been reported with olanzapine, ziprasidone, quetiapine and zotepine. Despite a number of methodological problems, early results suggest that this is another potential advantage for the new-generation antipsychotic medications. The degree to which these medications will improve functional outcome remains to be seen.

Alternative strategies

It may be simplistic to assume that one medication will be maximally effective in alleviating positive, negative and cognitive symptoms. Therefore, there will be increasing research on adjunctive treatments that might enhance cognitive functioning, but as yet there are no proven safe and effective treatments.

Studies of cognitive remediation strategies in schizophrenia have shown some encouraging results.[149,150] Future research in this area may lead to new clinical strategies.

Psychosocial management strategies

Although pharmacologic treatment is fundamental to the management of schizophrenia, psychosocial interventions are also necessary to ensure optimum outcome and functional adaptation. A variety of interventions have been studied, ranging from cognitive remediation and cognitive behaviour therapy to family therapy, psychoeducation, social skills training and vocational rehabilitation. There is often overlap in the design and application of these strategies.

The Schizophrenia Patient Outcomes Research Team recommendations for the treatment of schizophrenia, based on scientific evidence and exhaustive reviews of the literature, are outlined in Table 14. As further knowledge is gained about specific domains of deficits in schizophrenia, it is hoped that more specific, targeted approaches to both biologic and psychosocial interventions can be developed.

Table 14 *Schizophrenia Patient Outcomes Research Team recommendations for the treatment of schizophrenia.*[128]

Psychological treatments	Individual and group psychotherapies adhering to a psychodynamic model (defined as therapies that use interpretation of unconscious material and focus on transference and regression) should not be used in the treatment of persons with schizophrenia. Individual and group therapies employing well-specified combinations of support, education and behavioural and cognitive skills training approaches designed to address the specific deficits of persons with schizophrenia should be offered over time to improve functioning and enhance other targeted problems, such as medication non-compliance.
Family treatments	Patients who have ongoing contact with their families should be offered a family psychosocial intervention that spans at least 9 months and provides a combination of education about the illness, family support, crisis intervention and problem-solving skills training. Such interventions should also be offered to non-family caregivers. Family interventions should not be restricted to patients whose families are identified as having high levels of 'expressed emotion' (criticism, hostility, overinvolvement). Family therapies based on the premise that family dysfunction is the aetiology of the patient's schizophrenic disorder should *not* be used.

Table 14 *Contd.*

Vocational rehabilitation	Persons with schizophrenia who have any of the following characteristics should be offered vocational services: The person (a) identifies competitive employment as a personal goal, (b) has a history of prior competitive employment, (c) has a minimal history of psychiatric hospitalization, and (d) is judged on the basis of a formal vocational assessment to have good work skills. The range of vocational services available in a service system for persons with schizophrenia living in the community who meet the criteria defined above should Include (a) prevocational training, (b) transitional employment, (c) supported employment, and (d) vocational counselling and education services (job clubs, rehabilitation counselling, post-employment services).
Services systems	Systems of care serving persons with schizophrenia who are high services users should include assertive case management and assertive community treatment programs. Assertive community treatment programs should be targeted to individuals at high risk for repeated rehospitalizations or who have been difficult to retain in active treatment with more traditional types of services.

References

1 World Health Organization. *International Classification of Diseases*, 10th edn (ICD-10). Geneva: WHO, 1994.

2 American Psychiatric Association. *Diagnostic and Statistical Manual of Mental Disorders*, 4th edn (DSM-IV). Washington, DC: American Psychiatric Press, 1994.

3 Endicott J, Spitzer RL. A diagnostic interview: the schedule for affective disorders and schizophrenia (SADS). *Arch Gen Psych* 1978;**35**:837–844.

4 Spitzer RL, Williams JD, Gibon M, First MB. *Structured clinical interview for DSM-III–R-SCID*. Washington, DC: American Psychiatric Press, 1990.

5 World Health Organization. *Composite International Diagnostic Interview* (CIDI) 1.1 ed. Geneva: WHO, 1994.

6 Carpenter WT Jr, Heinrichs DW, Alphs LD. Treatment of negative symptoms. *Schizophr Bull* 1985;**11**:440–452.

7 Walker EF, Grimes KE, Davis DM, et al. Childhood precursors of schizophrenia: facial expressions of emotion. *Am J Psych* 1993;**150**:1654–1660.

8 Jones P, Rodgers B, Murray R, et al. Child development risk factors for adult schizophrenia in the British 1946 birth cohort. *Lancet* 1994;**344**:1398–1402.

9 Parnas J, Cannon TD, Jacobson B, et al. Lifetime DSM-III-R diagnostic outcomes in the offspring of schizophrenic mothers. Results from the Copenhagen high-risk study. *Arch Gen Psych* 1993;**50**:707–714.

10 Loebel AD, Lieberman JA, Alvir JM, et al. Duration of psychosis and outcome in first-episode schizophrenia. *Am J Psych* 1992;**149**:1183–1188.

11 Craig TJ, Bromet EJ, Fennig S, et al. Is there an association between duration of untreated psychosis and twenty-four month

clinical outcome in a first admission series? *Am J Psych* 2000;**157**:60–66.
12 Barnes TRE, Hutton SB, Chapman MJ, et al. West London first-episode study of schizophrenia: clinical correlates of duration of untreated psychosis. *Br J Psych* 2000; (in press).
13 May PR, Tuma AH, Yale C, et al. Schizophrenia — a follow-up study of results of treatment. II. Hospital stay over two to five years. *Arch Gen Psych* 1976;**33**(4):481–486.
14 Falloon IRH, Kydd RR, Coverdale JH, Laidlaw TM. Early detection and intervention for initial episodes of schizophrenia. *Schizophr Bull* 1996;**22**:271–282.
15 McGorry PD, Edwards J, Mihalopoulos C, et al. EPPIC: an evolving system of early detection and optimal management. *Schizophr Bull* 1996;**22**:305–326.
16 Larsen TK, Johannessen JO, Opjordsmoen S. First episode schizophrenia with long duration of untreated psychosis. *Br J Psych* 1998;**172**:45–52.
17 Cornblatt B. Predictors of schizophrenia and preventive intervention. In Breier A, Tran PV, Bymaster R and Tollefson C (eds) *Current Issues in the Psychopharmacology of Schizophrenia.* Williams & Wilkins, 2000.
18 Allison DB, Mentore JL, Moonseong H, et al. Antipsychotic-induced weight gain: a comprehensive research synthesis. *Am J Psychiatr* 1999;**56**:1686–1696.
19 Haffner H, Maurer K, Loffler W, Riecher-Rossler A. The influence of age and sex on the onset and early course of schizophrenia. *Br J Psych* 1993;**162**:80–86.
20 Lieberman JA, Alvir JM, Koreen A, et al. Psychobiologic correlates of treatment response in schizophrenia. *Neuropsychopharmacology* 1996;**14**:13s–21s.
21 Ciompi L. The natural history of schizophrenia in the long term. *Br J Psych* 1980;**136**:413–420.
22 Hegarty JD, Baldessarini RJ, Tohen M, et al. One hundred years of schizophrenia: A meta-analysis of the outcome literature. *Am J Psych* 1994;**151**:1409–1416.
23 Kane JM, Honigfeld G, Singer J, Meltzer H and The Clozaril Collaborative Study Group. Clozapine for the treatment-resistant schizophrenic: a double-blind comparison with chlorpromazine. *Arch Gen Psych* 1988;**45**: 789–796.

24 Klein DF, Davis JM. *Diagnosis and Drug Treatment of Psychiatric Disorders*. Baltimore: Williams & Wilkins, 1969.
25 Janicak PG, Davis JM, Preskorn SH, Ayd FJ Jr. *Principles and Practice of Psychopharmacotherapy*. Baltimore: Williams & Wilkins, 1993.
26 Scatton B, Claustre Y, Cudennec A, et al. Amisulpride: from animal pharmacology to therapeutic action. *Int Clin Psychopharm* 1997;**12**(suppl. 2):S29–S36.
27 Puech A, Fleurot O, Rein W. Amisulpride, an atypical antipsychotic, in the treatment of acute episodes of schizophrenia: a dose-ranging study vs haloperidol. The Amisulpride Study Group. *Acta Psychiatr Scand* 1998;**98**:65–72.
28 Freeman HL. Amisulpride compared with standard neuroleptics in acute exacerbations of schizophrenia: three efficacy studies. *Int Clin Psychopharmacol* 1997;**12**(suppl 2):S11–S117.
29 Moller HJ, Boyer P, Fleurot O, Rein W. Improvement of acute exacerbations of schizophrenia with amisulpride: a comparison with haloperidol. PROD-ASLP study group. *Psychopharmacology* (Berl) 1997;**132**: 396–401.
30 Wetzel H, Gründer E, Hillert A, et al. Amisulpride versus flupentoxil in schizophrenia with predominantly positive symptomatology – a double-blind controlled study comparing a selective D_2-like antagonist to a mixed D_1-/D_2- like antagonist. *Psychopharmacol* 1998;**137**:223–232.
31 Chouinard G, Jones B, Remington G, et al. A Canadian multi center placebo-controlled study of fixed doses of risperidone and haloperidol in the treatment of chronic schizophrenic patients. *J Clin Psychopharmacol* 1993;**13**:25–40.
32 Marder SR, Meibach RC. Risperidone in the treatment of schizophrenia. *Am J Psych* 1994;**151**:825–835.
33 Flynn SW, MacEwan GW, Altman S, et al. An open comparison of clozapine and risperidone in treatment-resistant schizophrenia. *Pharmacopsychiatry* 1998;**31**:25–29.
34 Bondolfi G, Dufour H, Patris M, et al. Risperidone versus clozapine in treatment-resistant chronic schizophrenia: a randomized double-blind study. *Am J Psych* 1998;**155**:499–504.
35 Schooler N, Marder S, Kane J, et al. Clozapine and risperidone: a 29 week randomized clinical trial. *Schizophr Res* 1999;**36**:296.
36 Bymaster FP, Calligaro DO, Falcone JF, et al. Radioreceptor binding profile of the atypical antipsychotic olanzapine. *Neuropsychopharmacology* 1996;**14**:87–96.

37 Beasley CM, Tollefson G, Tran P, et al. Olanzapine versus placebo and haloperidol: acute phase results of the North American double-blind olanzapine trial. *Neuropsychopharmacology* 1996;**14**:111–123.
38 Tollefson GD, Beasley CM, Tran P. Olanzapine versus haloperidol in the treatment of schizophrenia and schizoaffective and schizophreniform disorders: results of an international collaborative trial. *Am J Psych* 1997;**154**:457–465.
39 Tollefson GD, Sanger TM, Lu Y, et al. Depressive signs and symptoms in schizophrenia: A prospective blinded trial of olanzapine and haloperidol. *Arch Gen Psych* 1998;**55**:250–258.
40 Tran PV, Hamilton SH, Kuntz HA, et al. Double-blind comparison of olanzapine versus risperidone in the treatment of schizophrenia and other psychotic disorders. *J Clin Psychopharm* 1997;**17**:407–418.
41 Martin J, Gomez JC, Garcia-Bernardo E, et al. Olanzapine and treatment-refractory schizophrenia: results of an open-label study. *J Clin Psych* 1997;**58**:479–491.
42 Baldacchino AM, Stubbs JH, Nevison-Andrews D. The use of olanzapine in non-compliant or treatment-resistant clozapine populations in hospital. *Pharmaceut J* 1998;**260**:207–209.
43 Breier A, Hamilton SH. Comparative efficacy of olanzapine and haloperidol for patients with treatment-resistant schizophrenia. *Biolog Psych* 1999;**45**: 403–410.
44 Conley RR, Tamminga CA, Bartko JJ, et al. Olanzapine compared with chloropromazine in treatment-resistant schizophrenia. *Am J Psych* 1998;**155**:914–920.
45 Small JG, Hirsch SR, Arvanitis LA, et al. Seroquel Study Group. Quetiapine in patients with schizophrenia: a high- and low-dose double-blind comparison with placebo. *Arch Gen Psych* 1997;**54**:549–557.
46 Arvanitis LA, Miller DG and the Seroquel Trial Thirteen Study Group. Multiple fixed doses of 'Seroquel' (quetiapine) in patients with acute exacerbation of schizophrenia: a comparison with haloperidol and placebo. *Biol Psychiatr* 1997;**42**:233–246.
47 Peuskens J, Linck CG. A comparison of quetiapine and chloropromazine in the treatment of schizophrenia. *Acta Psychiatr Scand* 1997;**96**:265–273.

48 Glazer WM, Morgenstern H, Pultz JA, et al. Quetiapine-tardive dyskinesia? Poster presented at American College of Neuropsychopharmacology, Acapulco, Mexico, 12–16 December 1999.
49 Emsley RA, Raniwalla J, Bailey TJ, et al. Efficacy and tolerability of seroquel compared with haloperidol and schizophrenic patients partially responsive to conventional antipsychotic treatment. *Int Clin Psychopharmacol* 2000; (in press).
50 Zimbroff DL, Kane JM, Tamminga CA, et al. A controlled, dose-response study of sertindole and haloperidol in the treatment of schizophrenia. *Am J Psych* 1997;**154**:782–791.
51 VanKammen D, McEvoy J, Targum S, et al. A randomized, controlled, dose ranging trial of sertindole in patients with schizophrenia. *Psychopharmacology* 1996;**124**:168–175.
52 Daniel DG, Wozniak P, Mack RJ, et al. Long term efficacy and safety comparison of sertindole and haloperidol in the treatment of schizophrenia. *Psychopharmacol Bull* 1998;**34**:61–69.
53 Keck P Jr., Buffenstein A, Ferguson J, et al. Ziprasidone 40 and 120 mg/day and the acute exacerbation of schizophrenia and schizoaffective disorder: a four-week placebo-controlled trial. *Psychopharmacology* 1998;**140**:173–184.
54 Daniel DG, Zimbroff DL, Potkin SG, et al. Ziprasidone 80 mg/day and 160 mg/day in the acute exacerbation of schizophrenia and schizoaffective disorder: a six-week placebo-controlled trial. *Neuropsychopharmacology* 1999;**20**:490–505.
55 Hirsch S, Power A, Kissling W. Ziprasidone versus haloperidol in stable schizophrenia. Poster presented at 11th World Congress of Psychiatry, Hamburg, Germany, August 1999.
56 Arato M, O'Connor R, Meltzer H, Bradberry J. Ziprasidone: efficacy and the prevention of relapse and in the long-term treatment of negative symptoms of chronic schizophrenia. *Eur Psychopharm* 1997;**7**(suppl. 2):214.
57 Petit M, Raniwalla J, Tweed J, et al. A comparison of an atypical and typical antipsychotic, zotepine versus haloperidol in patients with acute exacerbation of schizophrenia: A parallel-group double-blind trial. *Psychopharmacol Bull* 1996;**32**:81–87.
58 Fleischhacker WW, Barnas C, Stuppack CH, et al. Zotepine versus haloperidol in paranoid schizophrenia: a double-blind trial. *Psychopharm Bull* 1989;**25**:97–100.

59 Klieser E, Lehmann E, Tegeler J. Double-blind comparison of three times 75 mg zotepine and three times 4 mg haloperidol in acute schizophrenics. *Fortschr Neurol Psychiatr* 1991;14–17.
60 Cooper SL, Butler A, Tweed J, et al. Zotepine and the prevention of relapse. Poster presented at Sixth World Congress of Biological Psychiatry, Nice, France, 22–27 June 1997.
61 Barnas C, Stuppack CH, Miller C, et al. Zotepine in the treatment of schizophrenic patients with prevailingly negative symptoms. A double-blind trial vs haloperidol. *Int Clin Psychopharmacol* 1992;**7**:23–27.
62 Johnstone EC, Crow TJ, Johnson AL and MacMillan JF. The Northwick Park Study of first-episode schizophrenia: I. Presentation of the illness and problems relating to admission. *Br J Psych* 1986;**148**:115–120.
63 Birchwood M and MacMillan JF. Early intervention in schizophrenia. *Austr NZ J Psych* 1993;**27**:374–378.
64 Haas GL, Sweeney JA. Premorbid and onset features of first episode schizophrenia. *Schizophr Bull* 1992;**18**:373–386.
65 Beiser M, Erickson D, Fleming JAE, Iacono WG. Establishing the onset of psychotic illness. *Am J Psych* 1993;**150**:1349–1354.
66 McGorry PD and Singh BS. Schizophrenia: risk and possibility. In: Raphael B, Burrows GD (eds). *Handbook of Studies on Preventive Psychiatry*. Amsterdam: Elsevier, 1995: 491–514.
67 Chakos MH, Alvir JMP, Woerner MG, et al. Incidence and correlates of tardive dyskinesia in first episode in schizophrenia. *Arch Gen Psych* 1996;**53**:313–319.
68 Jeste DV, Okamoto A, Napolitano J, Kane JM, Martinez R. Low incidence of tardive dyskinesia in elderly patients with dementia treated with risperidone. *Am J Psych* 2000; (in press).
69 Kopala LC, Kimberley PG, Honer WG. Extrapyramidal signs and clinical symptoms in first episode schizophrenia: response to low-dose risperidone. *J Clin Psychopharmacol* 1997;**17**:308–313.
70 Farde L, Nordstrom AL, Wiesel FA. Positron admission tomographic analysis of central D_1 and D_2 dopamine receptor occupancy in patients treated with classical neuroleptics and clozapine. *Arch Gen Psych* 1992;**49**:538–544.
71 Kinon BJ, Kane JM, Johns C, et al. Treatment of neuroleptic resistant schizophrenic relapse. *Psychopharm Bull* 1993;**29**(2):309–314.

72 Kane JM, Rifkin A, Quitkin F, Nayak DV, Ramos-Lorenzi JR. Fluphenazine versus placebo in patients with remitted, acute first episode schizophrenia. *Arch Gen Psych* 1982;**39**:70–73.
73 Crow TJ, MacMillan JF, Johnson AL, et al. The Northwick Park study of first episodes of schizophrenia II: a randomized controlled trial of prophylactic neuroleptic treatment. *Br J Psych* 1986;**148**:120–127.
74 American Psychiatric Association. Practice guideline for the treatment of patients with schizophrenia. *Am J Psych* 1997;**154**(4 suppl.):1–63.
75 McEvoy JP, Weiden PJ, Smith TE, et al. Expert consensus guidelines series: treatment of schizophrenia. *J Clin Psych* 1996;**57**(suppl. 12B):1–58.
76 Rabiner CJ, Wegner JT, Kane JM. Outcome study of first-episode psychosis. I: Relapse rates after one year. *Am J Psych* 1986;**143**: 1155–1158.
77 Prudo R, Blum M. Five year outcome and prognosis in schizophrenia. *Br J Psych* 1987;**150**:345–354.
78 McCreadie RG, Wiles D, Grant SM, Moore J. The Scottish first-episode schizophrenia study: V. One year follow up. *Br J Psych* 1988;**152**:470–476.
79 McCreadie RG, Livingston MG, Todd NA, et al. The Scottish first-episode schizophrenia study. VIII: Five-year follow up: Clinical and psychosocial findings. *Br J Psych* 1992;**161**:496–500.
80 Rajkumar S, Thara R. Factors effecting relapse in schizophrenia. *Schiz Res* 1989;**2**:403–409.
81 Zhang M, Wang M, Li J, Phillips MR. Randomized-control trial of family intervention for seventy eight first-episode male schizophrenia patients. An eighteen month study in Suzhou, Jiangsu. *Br J Psych* 1994;**165**(suppl. 24):96–102.
82 Linszen DH, Dingemans PM, Lenior ME. Cannabis abuse and the course of recent-onset schizophrenic disorders. *Arch Gen Psych* 1994;**51**:273–279.
83 Robinson D, Woerner MG, Alvir JM, et al. Predictors of relapse following response from a first episode of schizophrenia or schizoaffective disorder. *Arch Gen Psych* 1999;**56**:241–247.
84 Steingard S, Allen M, Schooler NR. A study of the pharmacologic treatment of medication compliant schizophrenics who relapse. *J Clin Psychiatry* 1994;**55**:470–472.

85 Kane JM, Woerner M, Borenstein M, Wegner J, Lieberman J. Integrating incidence and prevalence of tardive dyskinesia. *Psychopharm Bull* 1986;**22**:254–258.
86 Woerner MG, Alvir JM, Saltz B, Lieberman J, Kane JM. Prospective study of tardive dyskinesia in the elderly: rates and risk factors. *Am J Psych* 1998;**155**:1521–1528.
87 Umbricht DSG, Pollack S, Kane JM. Clozapine and weight gain. *J Clin Psych* 1994;**55**(suppl. B):157–160.
88 Hagg S, Joelsson L, Mjorndal T, et al. Prevalence of diabetes and impaired glucose tolerance in patients treated with clozapine compared with patients treated with conventional depot neuroleptic medications. *J Clin Psych* 1998;**59**:294–299.
89 Hirsch SR, Barnes TRE. Clinical use of high-dose neuroleptics. *Br J Psych* 1994;**164**:94–96.
90 Thompson C. The use of high-dose antipsychotic medication. *Br J Psych* 1994;**164**:448–458.
91 Pollack RB, Kane JM. Clozapine reduces rehospitalization among schizophrenia patients. *Psychopharm Bull* 1998;**34**:89–92.
92 Essock SM, Hargreaves WA, Covell NH, Goether J. Clozapine's effectiveness for patients in state hospitals: results from a randomized trial. *Psychopharm Bull* 1996;**32**:683–697.
93 Perry PJ, Miller DD, Arndt SV, et al. Clozapine and norclozapine plasma concentrations and clinical response of treatment-refractory schizophrenic patients. *Am J Psych* 1991;**148**:231–235.
94 Potkin SG, Bera R, Gulasekeram B, et al. Plasma clozapine concentrations predict clinical response in treatment-resistant schizophrenia. *J Clin Psych* 1994;**55**(suppl. 9):133–136.
95 Kronig MH, Munne RA, Szymanski S, et al. Plasma clozapine levels and clinical response for treatment-refractory schizophrenic patients. *Am J Psych* 1995;**152**: 179–182.
96 Friedman J, Ault K, Powchik P. Pimozide: Pimozide augmentation for the treatment of schizophrenic patients who are partial responders to clozapine. *Biolog Psych* 1997;**42**:522–523.
97 Henderson DC, Goff DC. Risperidone as an adjunct to clozapine therapy in chronic schizophrenics. *J Clin Psych* 1996;**57**:395–397.
98 Shiloh R, Zemishlany Z, Aizenberg D, et al. Sulpiride augmentation in people with schizophrenia partially responsive to clozapine. A double-blind, placebo-controlled study. *Br J Psych* 1997;**171**:569–573.

99 Mowerman S, Siris SG. Adjunctive loxapine in a clozapine-resistant cohort of schizophrenic patients. *Ann Clin Psych* 1996;**8**:193–197.
100 Small JG, Kellams JJ, Milstein V, et al. A placebo-controlled study of lithium combined with neuroleptics in chronic schizophrenic patients. *Am J Psych* 1975;**132**:1315–1317.
101 Growe GA, Crayton JW, Klass DB, et al. Lithium in chronic schizophrenia. *Am J Psych* 1979;**136**:454–455.
102 Carmen JS, Bigelow LB, Wyatt RJ. Lithium combined with neuroleptics in chronic schizophrenic and schizoaffective patients. *J Clin Psych* 1995;**42**:124–128.
103 Wilson WH. Addition of lithium to haloperidol in non-affective, antipsychotic non-responsive schizophrenia: a double blind, placebo controlled, parallel design clinical trial. *Psychopharmacology* 1993;**111**:359–366.
104 Terao T, Oga T, Nozaki S, et al. Lithium addition to neuroleptic treatment in chronic schizophrenia: a randomized, double-blind, placebo-controlled, cross-over study. *Acta Psychiatr Scand* 1995;**92**:220–224.
105 Schulz CS, Thompson PA, Jacobs M, et al. Lithium augmentation fails to reduce symptoms in poorly responsive schizophrenic outpatients. *Jour Clin Psych* 1999;**60**:366–372.
106 Schulz SC, Kahn EM, Baker RW, et al. Lithium and carbamazepine augmentation in treatment-refractory schizophrenia. In: Angrist B, Schulz SC (eds.) *The Neuroleptic-Nonresponsive Patient: Characterization and Treatment.* Washington, DC: American Psychiatric Press, 1990: 109–136.
107 Arana GW, Goff DC, Friedman H, et al. Does carbamazepine-induced reduction of plasma haloperidol levels worsen psychotic symptoms? *Am J Psych* 1986;**143**:650–651.
108 Wolkowitz OM, Turetsky N, Reus VI, et al. Benzodiazepine augmentation of neuroleptics in treatment-resistant schizophrenia. *Psychopharm Bull* 1992;**28**: 291–295.
109 Ruskin P, Averbukh I, Belmaker RH, et al. Benzodiazepines in chronic schizophrenia. *Biolog Psych* 1979;**14**:557–558.
110 Johns CA, Thompson JW. Adjunctive treatments in schizophrenia: pharmacotherapies and electroconvulsive therapy. *Schizophr Bull* 1995;**21**:607–619.
111 Siris SG, Bermanzohn PC, Mason SE, et al. Maintenance imipramine therapy for secondary depression in schizophrenia: a controlled trial. *Arch Gen Psych* 1994;**51**:109-115.

112 Evins AE, Goff DC. Adjunctive antidepressant drug therapies in the treatment of negative symptoms. *CNS Drugs* 1996;**6**:130–147.
113 Fink M, Sackeim HA. Compulsive therapy in schizophrenia? *Schizophr Bull* 1996;**22**: 27–39.
114 Safferman AZ, Munne R. Case report combining clozapine with ECT. *Convul Ther* 1992;**8**:141–143.
115 Petrides G, Mendelowitz A, Fink M, Schooler N. ECT in clozapine resistant schizophrenia. Poster presentation, NCDEU Annual Meeting, Boca Raton, Florida, June 1999.
116 Chanpattana W, Chakrabhand S, Kongsakom R, et al. The short term effect of combined ECT and neuroleptic therapy in therapy persistent schizophrenia. *Convuls Ther* 2000; (in press).
117 Davis JM. Overview: maintenance therapy in psychiatry: I. Schizophrenia. *Am J Psych* 1975;**132**:1237–1245.
118 Kane JM, Lieberman JA. Maintenance pharmacotherapy in schizophrenia. In: Meltzer HY (ed) *Psychopharmacology: The Third Generation of Progress*. New York, Raven Press, 1103–1109, 1987.
119 Gilbert PL, Harris NJ, McAdams LA, Jeste DV. Neuroleptic withdrawal in schizophrenic patients: review of the literature. *Arch Gen Psych* 1995;**52**:173–188.
120 Kane JM, Smith J. Tardive dyskinesia: Prevalence and risk factors – 1959–1979. *Arch Gen Psych* 1982;**39**:473–481.
121 Kane JM. Tardive dyskinesia: epidemiological and clinical presentation. In Bloom FE and Kupfer DJ (eds) *Psychopharmacology: The Fourth Generation of Progress*. New York, Raven Press, 1485–1496, 1995.
122 Saltz BL, Woerner MG, Kane JM, et al. Prospective study of tardive dyskinesia incidence in the elderly. *JAMA* 1991;**266**:2402–2406.
123 Jeste DV, Caligiuri MP, Paulsen JS, et al. Risk of tardive dyskinesia in older patients: A prospective longitudinal study of 266 outpatients. *Arch Gen Psych* 1995;**52**:756–765.
124 Glazer WM, Kane JM. Depot neuroleptic therapy: an underutilized treatment option. *J Clin Psych* 1992;**53**(12):426–433.
125 Kemp R, Kirov G, Everitt B, et al. Randomized controlled trial of compliance therapy: 18 month follow up. *Br J Psych* 1998;**172**:413–419.
126 Fenton WS, Blyler CR, Heinssen RK. Determinants of medication compliance in schizophrenia: Empirical and clinical findings. *Schizophr Bull* 1997;**23**:637–651.

127 Robinson D, Woerner M, Alvir JM, Goldman R, Lieberman JA. Characteristics of patients with first episode schizophrenia who later become non-compliant with antipsychotics. ACNP Annual Meeting, Puerto Rico, 1998.
128 Lehman AF, Steinwachs DM, et al. Translating research into practice: the Schizophrenia Patient Outcomes Research Team (PORT) treatment recommendations. *Schizophr Bull* 1998;**24**:1–10.
129 Kane JM. Treatment of schizophrenia. *Schizophr Bull* 1987;**13**: 133–156.
130 Kane JM, Rifkin A, Woerner M, et al. Low-dose neuroleptic treatment of outpatient schizophrenics. I. Preliminary results for relapse rates. *Arch Gen Psych* 1983;**40**:893–896.
131 Viguera AC, Baldessarini RJ, Hegarty JD, et al. Clinical risk following abrupt and gradual withdrawal of maintenance and neuroleptic treatment. *Arch Gen Psych* 1997;**54**:49–55.
132 Tollefson GD, Beasley CM Jr, Tamura RN, et al. Blind, controlled, long-term study of the comparative incidence of treatment-emergent tardive dyskinesia with olanzapine or haloperidol. *Am J Psych* 1997;**154**:1248–1254.
133 Tariot P, Salzman C, Yeung P, et al. Clinical improvement and tolerability is maintained long-term in elderly patients with psychotic disorders treated with quetiapine. Poster presented at American College of Neuropsychopharmacology Annual Meeting, Acapulco, Mexico, December 1999.
134 Chatterjee A, Chakos M, Koreen A, et al. Prevalence and clinical correlates of extrapyramidal signs and spontaneous dyskinesias in never medicated schizophrenic patients. *Am J Psych* 1995;**152**: 1724–1729.
135 Carman J, Peuskens J, Vangeneugden A. Risperidone in the treatment of negative symptoms of schizophrenic: a meta-analysis. *Int Clin Psychopharmacol* 1995;**10**:207–213.
136 Saletu B, Kufferle B, Grunberger J, et al. Clinical, EEG mapping and psychometric studies in negative schizophrenia comparative trials with amisulpride and fluphenazine. *Neuropsychobiology* 1994;**29**:125–135
137 Moller H-J, Muller H, Borinson RL, Schooler NR, Chouinard G. A path-analytical approach to differentiate between direct and indirect drug effects on negative symptoms in schizophrenic patients: A re-evaluation of the North American risperidone study. *Eur Arch Psych* 1995;**245**:45–49.

138 Siris SG, Adan F, Cohen M, et al. Post-psychotic depression and negative symptoms: an investigation of syndromal overlap. *Am J Psych* 1988;**145**:1532–1537.
139 Goff DC, Tsai G, Levitt J, et al. A placebo-controlled trial of d-cycloserine added to conventional neuroleptics in patients with schizophrenia. *Arch Gen Psych* 1999;**56**:21–27.
140 Javitt DC, Zylberman I, Zukin SR, et al. Amelioration of negative symptoms in schizophrenia by glycine. *Am J Psych* 1994;**151**:1234–1236.
141 Green MF. What are the functional consequences of neurocognitive deficits in schizophrenia? *Am J Psych* 1996;**153**:321–330.
142 Seidman LJ, Pepple JR, Faraone SV. Neuropsychological performance in chronic schizophrenia in response to neuroleptic dose reduction. *Biolog Psych* 1993;**33**:575–584.
143 Keefe SE, Perkins D, Silva SM, Lieberman JA. The effect of atypical antipsychotic drugs on neurocognitive impairment in schizophrenia: a review and meta-analysis. *Schizophr Bull* 1999;**25**:201–222.
144 Velligan DI, Newcomer J, Pultz J, et al. Improvement in cognitive functioning with long-term quetiapine is superior to haloperidol. Poster presented at American College of Neuropsychopharmacology Annual Meeting, Acapulco, Mexico, December, 1999.
145 Saykin AJ, Gur RC, Gur RE, et al. Neuropsychological function in schizophrenia: Selective impairment in memory and learning. *Arch Gen Psych* 1991;**48**:618–624.
146 Gold JM, Randolph C, Carpenter CJ, et al. Forms of memory failure in schizophrenia. *J Abnorm Psych* 1992;**101**:487–494.
147 Addington J, Addington D, Maticka-Tyndale E. Cognitive functioning and positive and negative symptoms in schizophrenia. *Schiz Res* 1991;**5**:123–134.
148 Harvey PD, Keefe SE. Cognition and new antipsychotics. *J Adv Schizophr Brain Res* 1998;**1**:2-8.
149 Wykes T, Reeder C, Corner J, et al. The effects of neurocognitive remediation on executive processing in patients with schizophrenia. *Schizophr Bull* 1999;**25**:291–307.
150 Spaulding WD, Fleming SK, Reed D, et al. Cognitive functioning in schizophrenia: Implications for psychiatric rehabilitation. *Schizophr Bull* 1999;**25**:275–289.

Index